GW00838472

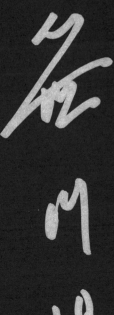

NO MATTER WHERE THE JOURNEY TAKES ME

YOHEI SASAKAWA

No Matter Where the Journey Takes Me

One Man's Quest for a Leprosy-free World

Translated by
Rei Muroji

HURST & COMPANY, LONDON

First published in the United Kingdom in 2019 by
C. Hurst & Co. (Publishers) Ltd.
41 Great Russell Street, London, WC1B 3PL
©Yohei Sasakawa, 2019
All rights reserved.
Printed in the United Kingdom by Bell & Bain Ltd, Glasgow

The right of Yohei Sasakawa to be identified as the author of
this publication is asserted by him in accordance with the
Copyright, Designs and Patents Act, 1988.

Distributed in the United States, Canada and Latin America by
Oxford University Press, 198 Madison Avenue, New York, NY 10016,
United States of America.

A Cataloguing-in-Publication data record for this book is available
from the British Library.

ISBN: 9781787381377

This book is printed using paper from registered sustainable
and managed sources.

www.hurstpublishers.com

CONTENTS

PREFACE

My first encounter with Yohei Sasakawa dates back almost thirty years to when I was an epidemiologist from the US Centers for Disease Control working for the World Health Organization (WHO) in the area of communicable disease control. Prior to this I had worked for two years on the smallpox eradication programme in India, and as a result saw first-hand the benefits of a global effort to rid the world of a greatly feared and devastating infectious disease. It was during this period, and also during a subsequent twelve-year assignment to ministries of health in sub-Saharan Africa, that I became aware of the high prevalence of, and severe disability and social discrimination being caused by leprosy. It was only natural, then, that when the generous and devoted efforts of Mr. Yohei Sasakawa to mobilize the world towards the elimination of leprosy came fully to my attention (and admiration) at WHO, I would strive to learn more about this man and his dedication. In *No Matter Where the Journey Takes Me*, Mr. Sasakawa describes much of what he told me as we discussed his life and mission together.

Mr. Sasakawa is a remarkable eighty-year-old Japanese philanthropist and social activist; in this book he lays out his personal mission and philosophy regarding the fight against leprosy. When we first met, he was president of the Nippon Foundation, and we often shared our thoughts about the importance of a unified global effort to eliminate leprosy, and of the need to decrease the many leprosy-related stigmas and the resulting discrimination. In particular I was fascinated to learn how Mr. Sasakawa had become engaged in this effort because of the influence of his father, Ryoichi Sasakawa, the founder of the Nippon Foundation, which since 1974 has provided over 200 million US dollars for leprosy control and elimination.

In *No Matter Where the Journey Takes Me*, Mr. Sasakawa describes how his father's compassion for those with leprosy began when he was a young man and had emotional feelings for a beautiful girl living in the village where he was born. Then, one day, this girl vanished: he later understood that her disappearance was because she had developed leprosy and had been sent to be isolated with others who had the same fate.

Mr. Sasakawa has often told me that because of his father's compassion, the elimination of leprosy has become his "destiny", just as it had been for his father. And the book he has written clearly demonstrates this. He first writes about how leprosy has been regarded by society since biblical times: incurable, dangerously infectious, unclean, and punishment for one's sins. As a result, patients were forcibly isolated and excluded from society under the law. But even after the discovery of effective ways to diagnose and treat leprosy in the early 1980s, the isolation, alienation and stigmatisation of many of those affected by leprosy did not end.

Having made visits to leprosy patients with his father, Mr. Sasakawa describes how he came to fully embrace his father's mission, and has ensured that the elimination of leprosy remains a major objective of the Nippon Foundation. He tells, for example, how during a five-year period between 1995 and 1999 the Nippon Foundation provided funding to the WHO, sufficient to pay for the medicine needed to cure those estimated to have leprosy worldwide. He further describes how these medicines were then made available to countries so that they could be supplied at no cost to leprosy patients wherever they were found.

By providing leprosy medication at no cost, Mr. Sasakawa made it possible for all those with leprosy to have access to effective treatment. He also provided support for screening and early diagnosis of persons without symptoms so that they could be treated before disabilities occurred, and the stigma and discrimination that result from physical deformity were thus prevented. During the first five-year period of this medicine donation programme, approximately 5 million people were cured of leprosy.

By the end of 2000, the leprosy elimination programme of WHO had reached its global target of less than one person with leprosy for every 10,000 persons. It was at this time that the WHO formed the Global Alliance for the Elimination of Leprosy to better unify the efforts of governments and leprosy NGOs in order to more effectively continue the fight against leprosy worldwide.

Since 2004 Mr. Sasakawa has worked as an official WHO Goodwill Ambassador for Leprosy Elimination, and has visited more than ninety countries to meet with national leaders in order to continue to engage them in the fight against leprosy, and especially to convince them of the need for those who have lasting disabilities to be permitted to become productive members of society rather than remaining in isolation. He describes these country missions fully—from his travels to the remotest parts of India and the Democratic Republic of the Congo, to his meetings with heads of state to make them aware of the condition of those with leprosy and leprosy disability, and to champion their needs. Through a series of high-visibility global appeals for the rights of those with leprosy, Mr. Sasakawa succeeded in helping the world understand that leprosy discrimination is a human rights issue. His continued advocacy led the Japanese Government to introduce a draft resolution to the United Nations Human Rights Council (UNHRC) in 2008, calling for the elimination of discrimination and stigma against those affected by leprosy, and their family members; the resolution was adopted unanimously, and was subsequently adopted by the UN General Assembly in 2010.

No Matter Where the Journey Takes Me is the story of a man who has selflessly dedicated his life to bettering the lives of others by contributing to the elimination of leprosy, and by advocating the end of the social discrimination it causes. It is the story of a disfiguring disease that has afflicted humankind since before history was written, and of a man with a destiny and a mission who is making a difference.

David L. Heymann, M.D.

Professor of Infectious Disease Epidemiology,
London School of Hygiene and Tropical Medicine

Head of the Centre on Global Health Security at Chatham House, London

Chairman of Public Health England, United Kingdom

INTRODUCTION

"My life is my message."—Mahatma Gandhi
"I am my own witness."—Antoine de Saint-Exupéry, *Terres des hommes*

My Father's Legacy

There is a scene I will never be able to forget.

In the wee hours of 10 March 1945, amid the din of air raid sirens blaring in the darkness, formations of U.S. Army B-29 bombers appeared in the skies over Tokyo. At the time, I was six years old and living in what was then the Matsukiyo-cho area of Asakusa. My mother was racked with a high fever that had started the previous day, but I pulled her from her futon and together we fled from home. The streets were filled with people and handcarts, everyone chaotically rushing to escape from danger. That's when the incendiary bombs began raining down without mercy, and in no time the whole area was in flames, transforming the night into the illusion of daylight.

Amid the flames, people were writhing in agony, screaming in pain as the oil spilled from the firebombs rendered them all the more vulnerable to the blaze. Blackened corpses were strewn everywhere, heaped one upon the other. I nearly froze in my tracks, stunned by the horrific scene unfolding around me, but forced myself to keep moving, the air now scorching hot, making it difficult to breathe. My back was weighed down by a small bundle of rice—enough for my mother and I to survive for a week, and the only thing of value we had taken with us.

As we made our way in the direction of Ueno, we came to a Shinto shrine and my mother became unable to go any further. She sat herself down on the shrine's steps, "Run on without me," she gasped, "and have strength to live!" I looked around and saw a bicycle store that had so far escaped the fire. I ran in and asked for a cup of water for my mother. The proprietor was very kind, and let us stay the night inside his house. Without

1

the kindness we were shown that night, I'm sure my mother wouldn't have survived. I don't know what would have happened to me, just a young boy, either. In that one single night, Tokyo burned to the ground and more than 100,000 people lost their lives.

The next morning we returned to our home, only to find that everything had burned to ashes. All we found were two rice bowls, now melted together from the intense heat.

Higashi-Honganji Temple, not far away, had been turned into a temporary morgue. Whenever people who came looking for family members found the body of someone they knew, they would write the person's name on a scrap of paper and place it by the body. One body was that of an old woman who had died while holding her grandchild in her arms to protect him. I knew her. Her entire body was charred black, a pitiful sight, but to the very end she must have tried desperately to protect the child, for her grandson's body hadn't burned at all. It's a scene that still comes back to haunt me from time to time.

I have a destiny that I have to accept, and a mission that is of my own choosing.

My father was Ryoichi Sasakawa. He is a famous man, someone whom any Japanese who lived in the second half of the twentieth century would know of. Even now, more than twenty years after his death, much speculation and myriad misunderstandings abound concerning my father's outsize life as a political and social activist in the years of upheaval before and after World War II. And even today, at the age of eighty, I continue to be forever labelled "the son of Ryoichi Sasakawa".

I was born the illegitimate son of Ryoichi Sasakawa. I was raised by my mother. At the time of the "great" bombing of Tokyo—and both before and after—I lived in a home with no father. Other than the photograph my mother had placed on our Buddhist altar, I had no way of knowing this "father" of mine. Even when an unfamiliar man suddenly appeared in our home during my childhood, I was unable to recognize this perfect stranger as my "father."

When I was 15, I met my father for the first time, in my uncle's office in Osaka. He was better-looking than the person I had seen in that photograph, with clean, sharp features and a penetrating gaze. He suggested that I come to Tokyo, to study. I hesitated, for my mother was in poor health, my two elder brothers had already left home, and I didn't want to leave her on her own. But my mother wouldn't hear of it, and urged me to go. And so I left Osaka and moved to Tokyo, and began living together with my father. Father's "Tokyo wife"—his real wife was living in Osaka—was young and good-natured.

INTRODUCTION

As I got to know my father for the first time, and on close terms, I saw that he was always busy to an extreme degree. He was forever rushing about, assiduously attending to tasks all over the nation, from promoting motorboat racing to visiting disabled war veterans, to undertaking activities in support of a variety of causes. On those rare occasions when he was at home, he received a seemingly endless stream of visitors: war widows and others seeking his help in finding a job or dealing with their personal issues. As we had agreed, I spent my days going to school, and when not at school I helped clean and do chores around the house from early morning—and attend to my father's visitors until long into the night.

My status wasn't so much that of a son as a lodger or servant. My father and I never had any heart-to-heart talks, yet I never felt rebellious. Whenever I thought back on the destitute life I had had before, I was grateful just to have food on the table every day. But more than that, as time passed I came to embrace deep feelings of respect toward my father and the way he selflessly devoted himself to the many people who sought to rely on him.

Without hesitation, my father would invariably extend a helping hand to anyone in dire straits. To me, he became more than the father whose blood courses through my veins; I came to look up to him as a mentor who, by his own example, taught me how we should live as human beings. He taught me the meaning of compassion, the highest virtue of humanity as expounded in Oriental philosophy.

The Nippon Foundation, where I now serve as chairman, was originally founded by my father as the Japan Shipbuilding Industry Foundation (JSIF). The financial resources enabling the JSIF's creation came from motorboat racing,[1] a sport firmly established in Japan by my father. My father has often been labelled a right-wing "Class A" war criminal,[2] and his having headed

---

[1] The Nippon Foundation draws the funds needed to support its many projects from a portion of the gambling revenues generated from Japanese motorboat racing. Motorboat racing in Japan is a philanthropy-oriented enterprise, having been established in 1951 specifically to aid a maritime shipping industry that had been devastated in World War II. Under this unique system, the majority of the funds taken in by motorboat racing are returned to gamblers as winnings. However, a small percentage is earmarked for philanthropic purposes. This money is managed by the Foundation, which then selects projects that show great promise of affecting fundamental change.

[2] After Japan's defeat in World War II, Ryoichi Sasakawa was imprisoned for a time as a suspected "Class A" (crimes against peace) war criminal by the Allied Forces,

Japan's largest philanthropic association "funded by gambling" makes him sound like a shady fixer who ruled the dark underside of postwar Japan. But the father I knew from actually working by his side was a true humanitarian, a man who was driven to devote every ounce of his wisdom and passion, completely and selflessly, to the betterment of the world and all humanity. My father saw motorboat racing as one way for Japan, a nation roundly defeated in war, to contribute to world peace.

What my father sought throughout his life wasn't to amass wealth for himself, but rather to generate wealth to be used to the benefit of Japan and, by extension, the entire world. In that context, motorboat racing was the way he envisioned to save the hordes of the weak who were relegated to the "dark side" of Japanese society as the country sprinted headlong toward postwar recovery.

My father never placed one human being above another, nor did he believe that money could be regarded as pure or sullied. And although he was often misunderstood throughout his life, he consistently lived by the creed that Japan existed by virtue of the support it received from the rest of the world, and that he himself existed by virtue of the blessings he received from his country. In keeping with that creed, he elected to use the proceeds from motorboat racing to perform a wide array of humanitarian activities in nations everywhere. Today, at a time when activities in the public interest conducted at the private level have become highly touted, the methodology my father adopted is increasingly acquiring new appreciation for its outstanding social foresight.

Carrying on my father's work, along with leadership of the JSIF, isn't a mission bestowed on me by my father. My father was a believer in the old adage cautioning that one shouldn't bequeath "beautiful rice paddies" to one's offspring (because doing so will only render them indolent). Far from leaving me his assets, he didn't seek to pass leadership of Japan's biggest philanthropic organization on to me. Right to his very end, he never chose a successor.

On his deathbed, the only thing my father bequeathed to me was an exhortation to "work for the benefit of the world". It was to carry out those words, as well as my father's creed, that I chose of my own accord to take over his position at the JSIF: today's Nippon Foundation. But there was one more task

---

"first, for leading campaigns instigating aggression, nationalism and hostility against the United States. And second, for his continued vigorous activities in an organization that strongly impedes the development of democracy in Japan." He was subsequently released without trial.

INTRODUCTION

I believed I also had to fulfil: to clear the wholly unfounded stain on the name of Ryoichi Sasakawa, my father and my life's mentor. This was my destiny— and one more mission—as the son of Ryoichi Sasakawa.

Just as my father continued to fight, never turning his head, I aspire to be just like him, never turning my eyes away.

As chairman of the Nippon Foundation, what I, like my father, have focused on most is to give a helping hand, to extend a hand of salvation, to people in the direst of situations, people who have been left behind by contemporary society. In particular, the core focus of my many years of activity around the world has been to achieve the global elimination of leprosy—Hansen's disease—a challenge my father addressed with intense passion but ultimately failed to see accomplished during his lifetime.

Leprosy is one of the oldest known diseases in the history of mankind. Although the disease itself is almost never fatal, because of its disfiguring effects if left untreated—severely deformed hands, feet and face—leprosy has long been said to be divine punishment or a disease inflicted on its sufferer as a result of karma, causing it to be feared with dread the world over. It wasn't until Armauer Hansen (1841–1912), a Norwegian physician, discovered the bacilli that cause leprosy in 1873 that it became possible to take a scientific and medical approach toward the disease. The first breakthrough in treatment occurred in the 1940s with the use of the drug promine, but it was in the 1980s—more than a century after Dr. Hansen's discovery—that the introduction of the outstanding treatment used today, multidrug therapy, made leprosy an easily curable disease.

Nonetheless, in many nations, misinformation and prejudice toward leprosy pervasive throughout society have long impeded the advancement of proper medical policies toward the disease. Even today, there continue to be many people who endure dual suffering: that of the disease itself and of the discrimination toward those affected by it.

The first time I was drawn into the battle against leprosy was when I accompanied my father on a trip to Korea in 1965, during which we visited a local leprosy hospital. It was the very first time that I actually met a leprosy patient.

Lying in their beds, the patients welcomed my father all wearing matching blue clothes for the occasion. Many had severely deformed hands or feet or faces. But what shocked me more was, without exception, that they all failed to show any trace of human expression, as though they had long let the lifeblood drain from their bodies out of despair. I shuddered at the sight and was too petrified to move.

My father showed no trepidation whatsoever, and taking each patient's hand in his own, he spoke to them and offered them words of encouragement. I suddenly found myself overwhelmed with respect for my father. And it suddenly came to me what I was meant to do, myself, from then on. I wanted some day to devote myself, as my father did, to humanitarian activities—and especially leprosy. The experience of that day left an indelible mark in my memory.

The Fight against Leprosy

Even with an outstanding treatment method, working to eliminate leprosy is by no means an easy task. So long as leprosy patients continue to exist, the medicine has to reach them—even if it be in the most remote and isolated villages where there is no electricity or running water. Furthermore, many leprosy patients are not used to taking medicine, so they need to be educated in these matters. Indeed, poverty plays a major role in the spread of leprosy. Undertaking activities to combat leprosy in countries with such serious social issues is always a test of patience, persistence and passion.

In the context of leprosy, the word "elimination" often comes into play. As defined by the World Health Organization (WHO), "elimination" equates to a registered prevalence of less than one case per 10,000 of the population. Unfortunately, today, when the routes of infection remain unidentified and no preventive medicine has been developed, "eradication"—complete and total—of leprosy still defies possibility.

Nevertheless, so long as the disease can be detected early and patients treated at an early stage in their disease, then leprosy is no longer a disease to be feared. Early detection and early treatment with MDT means they can be completely cured, without leaving any physical disfigurations or impairments, just as with other common diseases. That said, in order to achieve the target of eliminating leprosy, ultimately it's necessary to deliver MDT free of charge to the farthest corners of the earth, no matter how big the obstacles.

Through the years I have visited and met with patients in leprosy hospitals and with people affected by leprosy living in colonies and sanatoriums all around the world. My overarching aim has been to confirm, with my own eyes, that MDT is reaching them. And just as my father always did, I too have always sought to encourage persons with leprosy by taking their hands in mine or putting my arm around their shoulders, no matter how serious their condition might be. Some of them look frightened simply by my getting close to them, for all their lives they have been shunned even by their own families, and rarely, if ever, have they known the warmth of another human being. What should I say to these wounded souls? On any number of occasions I have been shocked and horrified by the depth of darkness that surrounds leprosy. My fervent wish is to shine a ray of hope, as quickly as possible, into the lives of those who continue to suffer from this age-old scourge.

With that aspiration in mind, over the years, I have tried to meet directly with the leaders of less economically developed countries that are home to large numbers of leprosy patients. I have shaken their hands, spoken with them one on one, and stated my case in respect of leprosy.

Compared with illnesses such as HIV-AIDS, malaria or tuberculosis, each of which afflicts a great many people around the world, the number of patients afflicted with leprosy is altogether lower—and for that reason, leprosy tends to fall low on the agenda of issues of immediate concern to governments when forming their official health-related policies. This is why I have made a point of going to speak directly with the leaders of nations everywhere, to explain the true situation surrounding leprosy, and to urge them to work to resolve leprosy-related issues at a national level. Whenever such leaders have voiced a solid commitment to me on the matter, they have immediately passed the word on to their health ministry or persons in charge of leprosy issues, spurring them to action.

I have also always accorded prime importance to securing cooperation from the media. Measures for dealing with leprosy-related issues cannot score any measure of success so long as misinformation concerning the disease is allowed to persist: mistaken notions such as that leprosy is an affliction imposed by karma, or that it is hereditary, or that it is a highly contagious disease. Through use of the mass media, it is necessary to get the general public in countries everywhere to understand that leprosy is a curable disease and that effective treatment is available free of charge—and also to know that discrimination against leprosy patients is impermissible. Whenever I shake hands with or embrace a person affected by leprosy in the presence of the media, and this is shown on television or in the newspapers, I feel I am helping to dispel fears about the disease.

Another invaluable act is to always give robust encouragement to the health workers and social workers who work directly "on the front lines". This is where the issues needing to be addressed exist; yet it is also where measures to resolve those existing problems can be devised. We need to listen to what health and social workers say, and to feed that information back to the political leaders and health ministries of all countries.

Since the 1980s, upwards of 16 million leprosy patients have been cured and the number of countries where the disease is endemic has dropped dramatically. By April 2017, the number of nations, other than small island states, in which the elimination target had yet to be achieved had been reduced to only one: Brazil. Despite the great difficulties involved in getting to this point, this accomplishment owes most to the dedicated workers and supporters who, armed with professional knowledge and methods, have poured all-encompassing passion into their work. Surely the day is not far off when the long-awaited elimination of leprosy as a public health problem in every country will become a reality.

That said, achievement of "elimination" worldwide will not mark an end to our leprosy-related activities. We need to remain vigilant, keep collaborating, and find an effective way to break transmission of the disease until a leprosy-free world is realized. More than anything, the harsh reality remains that even now people affected by leprosy—who have been cured of the disease itself—are not accepted by society at large.

Leprosy, in addition to being a medical issue, is a human rights issue. In order to bring the battle that humanity has fought against leprosy to its final end, dealing with the human rights aspect of leprosy presents another major challenge.

I first took up the challenge of addressing leprosy as a human rights issue in 2003.

At my own initiative, I went to Geneva to bring the matter to the attention of what was then the United Nations Commission on Human Rights (UNCHR). After that body was reorganized as the United Nations Human Rights Council (UNHRC), I continued to plead for the elimination of the stigma and discrimination against leprosy patients, people affected by leprosy, and their family members. What I sought to do seemed as difficult as the proverbial camel passing through the eye of a needle, but with patience and persistence, in June 2008, at the suggestion of the Japanese Government, a UN resolution titled "Elimination of discrimination against persons affected by leprosy and their family members" was unanimously adopted by 59 countries. Happily, moreover, I succeeded in persuading China and Cuba, perennial opponents of any proposal made by Japan to the UNHRC, not only to agree to the proposal by the Japanese Government but also to become a joint sponsor.

This was followed by the resolution's passage, by the full complement of 192 nations, at the UN General Assembly in December 2010, along with approval of an accompanying set of principles and guidelines. In this way, the United Nations formally confirmed that leprosy is a human rights issue that demands the world's full attention. It was an epoch-making moment.

Of course, in order for measures aligned with the UN's guidelines to be implemented fully in nations everywhere, it would still be necessary—as in the case of leprosy as a medical issue—for there to be specific programmes, institutions and numerous cooperating partners.

I often compare the fight against leprosy to the two wheels of a motorcycle. Here, "liberation from the disease" and "liberation from stigma and discrimination" are the motorcycle's front and rear wheels, and both have to function properly in order for the motorcycle to advance. This is a message I have taken to the entire world.

To achieve this message's ultimate goal, with cooperation from global leaders of different spheres, on or near the last Sunday of each January—a date designated "World Leprosy Day"—I have organized a "Global Appeal" concerning discrimination toward leprosy.

I have also advocated that it is the people affected by leprosy themselves who should play the leading role in the fight against the stigma and discrimination they suffer, and at all times I have collaborated to the greatest extent in their activities. Many people affected by leprosy, stifled by their fear that if they were to raise their voices they would suffer added discrimination, have been compelled to live quiet and unobtrusive lives in remote locations or on small islands isolated from the general population. Especially in countries such as India, even after they have been cured of their disease they have no means of livelihood, so many are forced to eke out an existence by begging.

In recognition of their plight, I established the Sasakawa-India Leprosy Foundation (S-ILF). S-ILF offers people affected by leprosy microcredit loans to enable them to lead independent lives, and a scholarship programme has been created to enable children of leprosy-affected families to go to school.

Motivation for Writing This Book

As successor to the chairmanship of the Nippon Foundation—the third to hold this office after my father and Ayako Sono[3]—I have continuously kept up an arduous schedule of leprosy-related activities, including overseas visits and

---

[3] Ayako Sono (1931–) is a prominent writer of fiction and essays. She has written over forty novels and essays and was honoured as a Person of Cultural Merit in 2003. After the death of Ryoichi Sasakawa, she was appointed chairperson of the Nippon Foundation, a position she filled until 2005. She founded an NGO named JOMAS, Japan Overseas Missionaries Assistance Society, to help Japanese missionaries pursuing their calling abroad.

duties three to four months of each year. I have often been asked by the media, both Japanese and foreign, why I, a Japanese, take such pains and pour such passion into the pursuit of leprosy elimination. Up to now, I have offered little by way of response.

Born during wartime to a father whose whole life was the target of endless public criticism and censure, I have inevitably been influenced and affected by those circumstances. But for a long time I believed the time was not ripe for me to discuss such matters.

In recent years, however, several close friends whose opinions I deeply value and trust suggested to me that now, if ever, was the time to clarify and make known what has motivated me. The result is this book. Ever since I was a young man, I have always pondered how best to live my life, and in this volume I decided to describe in detail what, through the years, has driven me.

My life has been greatly influenced by the example set by my father. In the wake of Japan's defeat in war, my father worried deeply over the country's future and the prospects for world peace. He took it upon himself to debate these issues heatedly with the leaders of Japan, keeping up a vigorous pace fuelled by a selfless desire to bring benefit to others. To me, who had experienced the depths of privation and destruction as a boy during the war, my father also embodied the spirit of the many "good" Japanese who, even in the most turbulent of times after the war when the nation's very existence was in peril, remained virtuous, embraced lofty aspirations, and set out to achieve the mission at hand. And they approached that mission with fierce determination, a preparedness never to relent in pursuing their nation's future.

I in turn became driven by the determination to live my life with that same Japanese spirit. And with that spirit as my guide, I have run the course of my life, never letting up.

Through this book, my hope is that readers will come to understand the path that I and the Nippon Foundation have taken in the quest to eliminate leprosy and address its human rights issues, as well as the beliefs and methodologies that have taken us this far. I also hope that readers will be able to relate closely to the twist of fate that has inspired me, a Japanese, to address difficult issues faced by all humanity.

Finally, I also fervently hope that the example I have set as a human being might light a fire of ambition within tomorrow's generation to carry on activities like mine well into the future.

1

LEARNING THE TRUTH ABOUT LEPROSY

A Scourge Inflicted as "Divine Punishment"?

Leprosy isn't a disease confined to history books

How much do we know about Hansen's disease, the affliction more commonly known as leprosy? How much do people today know about its symptoms? From my personal experience I would say most young people today know very little about this disease and the symptoms that accompany it. People of an older generation—those in their fifties or sixties—likely know more about leprosy, and in most instances the image they have of it is a highly abstract notion of a frightening and incurable disease—but a disease relegated to the pages of history.

What surprises me most is that even among members of the medical profession there are people who readily admit to having no knowledge of leprosy, as though ignorance of this disease is nothing out of the ordinary. Medical specialists though they are, many implicitly believe that leprosy is a disease of the past, an illness that has long been eradicated from the planet.

Leprosy is by no means a disease of the past. True, in Japan new cases of leprosy are rare. But when we examine the picture from a global perspective, although the situation in Western countries is similar to that of Japan, even today new cases of leprosy are occurring in India, Asia, Africa, the Middle East and South America.

Leprosy is an infectious disease that develops from a bacillus called *Mycobacterium leprae*. The disease attacks the skin and peripheral nerves, the membranes lining the upper respiratory tract, and the eyes, among other areas. If left untreated, leprosy causes nerve damage that then gives rise to various complications. Muscles become paralysed, sensation is lost in the hands and feet, and eyesight deteriorates—conditions that cause leprosy patients to continually suffer injuries or burns. When other bacteria then invade these wounds, ulcers and festering sores develop, and ultimately parts of the body become deformed or are even lost, resulting in permanent disabilities.

The majority of people who conjure up an image of leprosy as a frightening disease derive their fear from the powerful impression left by these physical transformations. But changes of these kinds, it must be emphasized, are secondary symptoms attributable to the bacterial infections that commonly afflict leprosy patients; they are not caused by the leprosy bacillus itself. Even so, it can easily be imagined how, in an era when medical knowledge and skills were still sorely lacking, when, ignorant of the fact that leprosy is an infectious disease, no effective treatment had yet been discovered, this disease instilled immeasurable fear in people.

Leprosy's existence has been known worldwide since antiquity, and because it was uniformly believed that once it was contracted there was no cure and physical deformities and disabilities would inevitably ensue, throughout history leprosy was looked upon as a form of divine punishment for evil deeds committed in a "previous lifetime"—an affliction incurred by the workings of one's karma.

Fortunately, leprosy has today become a curable disease. The initial breakthrough came in the middle of the twentieth century with the drug promin, later replaced by dapsone. From the 1980s, this was superseded by multidrug therapy (MDT), an orally administered regimen of various drugs that has proven to be highly effective in curing the disease. So long as the disease is detected early and an MDT programme is initiated without delay, the patient normally suffers no visible physical deformities or disabilities.

Today we also know that while leprosy continues to exist, it is one of the least contagious of all diseases. The chances of catching a common cold are far higher than the probability of contracting leprosy. Moreover, the number of leprosy patients is overwhelmingly small compared with the number of sufferers of other diseases. Furthermore, unlike AIDS, tuberculosis or malaria, for example, leprosy is rarely fatal.

If all the above is true, then couldn't one reasonably conclude that leprosy is a disease of the past after all? Sadly not, for to do so would err greatly from the truth. For although leprosy has in fact become a curable disease, new cases continue to occur. Most significantly, the inaccurate knowledge, misunderstanding and prejudice surrounding leprosy, a disease that has been feared since time immemorial, continue to exist, along with the severe discrimination and social stigma they engender. It is these psychological impairments afflicting society that continue to cause suffering among both leprosy patients and those who have been cured of the disease but whose lives continue to be affected by it, whether physically, socially, economically or psychologically.

Unfortunately, there seems to be no wonder drug in existence capable of curing this social prejudice. Lamentably, moreover, this social prejudice is a contributing cause to the phenomenon of persons with the disease who go untreated in spite of there now being an effective treatment programme. Sufferers will often hide the very fact of their disease because they realize that once it became known they had contracted leprosy, they would become a target of cruel discrimination. As they thus refrain from stepping forward and being treated, their disease progresses, damage to their nerves increases, and disabilities set in. When these disabilities become apparent, the individual becomes a target of even greater social discrimination. Until this vicious cycle is broken, there can be no true resolution to the issues surrounding leprosy.

My aspiration in writing this book is to make you, the reader, aware of the discrimination that persons affected by leprosy have historically suffered and of the lives that they have been forced to live because of their disease. At the same time I also want you to know that now, at this very moment, there are places all around the world where discrimination against leprosy remains deeply entrenched.

Even when a patient is cured of leprosy itself, notions that fuel prejudice continue to abound. "Leprosy is a hereditary disease." "Leprosy is highly contagious." "Leprosy is incurable." "Leprosy is divine punishment." The result is that not only the patient but also the patient's family members are made to endure a range of social discriminations. Opportunities for education and marriage are taken from them, as are all means of earning a living, forcing them to live destitute lives as beggars. People living their lives in such circumstances continue to exist all around the world, even in the twenty-first century.

In January 2014 I met such a person during a visit to Indonesia—someone who had been banished from his community. I came across him on the island of Biak in Papua province. His name is Abia Rumbiak, and he was living in a tiny shack, about three metres square, far from his village. The shack barely provided Abia with shelter from the elements: here and there the walls had gaping holes, leaving Abia completely vulnerable to malaria-carrying mosquitoes. He lived there alone, sleeping on the bare earthen floor.

Abia's "home" was equipped with none of life's normal necessities, and the only thing keeping him alive was the meagre food a female relative brought to him. Even this didn't come every day, and Abia said there are often times when he goes to sleep hungry. Until he contracted leprosy at the age of fifteen, he worked as a fisherman. Now, with no work, all he can do is walk about the immediate vicinity, using a wooden oar from his days as a fisherman as a crutch. Otherwise, the rest of his time he spends inside the shack. "The days seem very long," he says, and surely that is so. Occasionally people from his village pass near his shack, but they always walk past ignoring him completely, shunning all eye contact.

I found myself unable to just leave Abia there like that, and I promised him that we would have dinner together. That evening I visited his shack again, this time with food and drinks in hand. "I came as I said I would," I greeted him. Abia smiled in return, a melancholy look in his eyes. He said he couldn't recall the last time he had eaten together with someone. Abia was about forty-eight years old, and thinking how very long he had lived in isolation from his community, all by himself, I was at a loss for words. Inside the shack, an enormous number of mosquitoes and moths were flying mercilessly about.

Banishment from his village. Fierce discrimination. Decades of a life of loneliness. Perhaps it's only natural that the expression etched on Abia's face and the look in his eyes are tinged by profound sorrow. And yet, to me it seemed that any intense emotions of bitterness or enmity toward the villagers who banished him had by now faded away. At the same time, the expression on Abia's face struck me as resembling something I was at a loss to identify immediately. It was only later that I realized that his expression—most of all, Abia's quiet gaze filled with sorrow—was very similar to that of a Buddhist monk who has endured many years of strict religious training and self-discipline.

Pondering how harsh such a life must be—the unjustifiable discrimination that had forced such long lonely years on him, having no choice but to accept that discrimination and loneliness, and doing so with the air of a buddha, and yet in reality having to live in loneliness—once again I found myself falling utterly silent.

Even today, all around the world, persons affected by leprosy suffer unjustifiable discrimination and are banished from their communities. Every time I meet someone who has been forced to live such a life in isolation, I am shocked as if struck by a sledgehammer, I am saddened, and I feel acutely conscious of my own powerlessness. But merely feeling pummelled to the ground won't change anything. What I can do—the only thing I must do—is never to lose my fighting spirit, and to continue my fight to eliminate leprosy and the discrimination that surrounds it.

In Japan too, the consequences of leprosy are still with us. In locations throughout the archipelago, there are still sanatoriums where patients formerly were isolated—and where they continue to live even after they have been completely cured of their disease, because their families refuse to live with them, leaving them with nowhere else to turn. According to recent figures, residents of the nation's former leprosariums today number close to 1,500. Nearly all of them are elderly.

The fight against the stigma of leprosy

For many years I have been involved in issues surrounding leprosy, carrying on the work started by my father, Ryoichi Sasakawa, who devoted himself vigorously to the eradication of this disease. Since his death I have striven to continue his legacy through a multitude of supportive activities conducted through two organizations: the Nippon Foundation and the Sasakawa Memorial Health Foundation (SMHF) [as of 1 April 2019 known as Sasakawa Health Foundation]. Above all, our most important task has been to ensure that treatment reaches leprosy patients everywhere, even in the most remote corners of the earth. To achieve this aim, we have formed strong partnerships with health organizations and NGOs (non-governmental organizations) across the globe. At the same time, for this same purpose we have for many years furnished significant financial support to the World Health Organization (WHO). Our efforts, I say with confidence, have had enormous impact.

Data shows that a total of more than 16 million leprosy patients have been cured of their disease since the 1980s, when MDT was introduced. The number of patients recorded each year has also declined dramatically: from 5 million in 1985 to 250,000 in 2000, to 210,000 cases in 2017. These achievements have been possible thanks in part to the support from the Nippon Foundation, which enabled the provision of MDT drugs, free of charge, to all countries and regions around the world between 1995 and 1999, and the continuing drug donations by Novartis thereafter.

The ability to achieve these impressive results in such a short time can be attributed to the role played by the WHO, which has set clear targets for the elimination of leprosy as a public health problem and has taken strategic steps toward attaining them.

Treating leprosy as a public health issue means that examinations and treatments applying to this disease could henceforth be carried out as routine medical services. Until recently, leprosy patients in virtually all countries were unable to receive treatment unless they went to a special hospital or care facility, a situation that has been a source of immeasurable anguish for patients. Also, since the distant past, being barred from undergoing examination at a general hospital itself exacerbated the prejudice and discrimination against leprosy patients. As a first step to enabling any person anywhere to

15

receive treatment by MDT, integration of such medical services became indispensable.

Thanks to these efforts, as of today only Brazil and some small island states have yet to achieve the leprosy elimination target at a national level. At a sub-national level, there are still many "hot spots" where the prevalence rate of leprosy remains high: for example, inner-city slums and difficult-to-access mountainous areas. Nevertheless, the fact that leprosy, a disease that has been feared since the very beginnings of human history, is slowly but surely being vanquished must rank as an achievement of which humankind can be proud.

In 2001 I was honoured to receive the designation by the WHO of Special Ambassador for the Global Alliance for the Elimination of Leprosy (GAEL). Since that time I have continuously stood in the front line of activities focused on achieving the targets set by the WHO and promoting its strategies, and for that reason, the achievements that have been made in such short time toward eliminating leprosy are a source of great personal joy. I am proud to have been able—in tandem with the WHO, the governments of nations around the world, the Nippon Foundation and the Sasakawa Memorial Health Foundation—to make a significant contribution toward resolving one of humankind's most difficult problems.

Before this great task is fully completed, however, much remains to be done.

Among communicable diseases, leprosy is a leading cause of disability. Although it is curable, there are an estimated 3 million people living with leprosy-related disabilities today because they contracted the disease before MDT became available, or because they were diagnosed late. Also, what is most regrettable is that even now new cases of leprosy are being detected all around the world, cases in which patients already have visible physical defor-mities or disabilities because they have been diagnosed late.

Why, despite the fact that an effective treatment, MDT, already exists, and that MDT is available free of charge, does a situation such as this continue?

I believe the answer is to be found in the "stigma" that is attached to this disease. In Christianity, the word "stigma" refers to the "sacred wounds" suf-fered by Jesus during his crucifixion. But originally stigma signified a mark burned or stamped into the skin of a criminal or slave. From this etymological beginning, stigma came to denote an attribute or symbol of a kind that is shunned by society, discriminated against, or considered to be heresy.

The first sociologist to focus on this issue was Erving Goffman (1922–1982). In his work *Stigma: Notes on the Management of Spoiled Identity* (1963), Goffman defines "stigma" as something in an individual that unavoidably

16

attracts the attention of those he or she encounters, causes them to turn away, and induces them to ignore other, favourable attributes—the individual being one who, if only the stigma were not present, would be accepted in normal social interactions without any problem.

Even when leprosy patients are completely cured, they suffer discrimination by dint of the physical stigma the disease has left them. What's more, even when the individuals have no visible disabilities, the fact that they had this disease itself becomes a stigma, causing them to be ostracized by society. Until the potential for such social discrimination disappears, there will likely be no end to sufferers of leprosy who make no attempt to be examined and thereby lose the opportunity for early treatment, resulting in the development of serious disabilities.

This is the reason why all along I have asserted that medical treatment alone is insufficient to deal with leprosy in the twenty-first century, and that this "stigma" must also be addressed. I have used the analogy of the two wheels of a motorcycle—the front wheel represents medical treatment by MDT, and the back wheel activities to end stigma and discrimination. And I have said that unless these two wheels turn smoothly at the same speed, there can be no arrival at the "destination". That "destination" of course is the realization of a world without leprosy, and without the stigma and discrimination that accompany this illness.

Wherever I have gone in the world, with whomever I have met, I have consistently conveyed three simple messages: that leprosy is curable, that treatment is free, and that it is wrong to discriminate. If I can spread these three messages until they become social norms, then those who contract this illness should be able to undergo examination and receive treatment with full peace of mind. It will, without question, also become easier to realize the early detection and early treatment that are so indispensable to eliminating leprosy. Only then, I believe, will leprosy become a "disease of the past" in the true sense, a disease that people need not fear.

The History of Discrimination against Leprosy and the Isolation of Patients

Did the history of human discrimination begin with leprosy?

Medically speaking, there are still some aspects of leprosy that defy our understanding. For example, leprosy's infection route—how the disease is transmitted from one person to another—has yet to be definitively ascertained. It is generally assumed that the infection spreads through close and frequent contact with an infected, untreated person. At the very least, we know that leprosy is not transmitted via a simple handshake or hug. Nearly everyone is born with a natural immunity to leprosy, so that even if we are exposed to the leprosy bacillus we do not come down with the disease.

Whenever I meet with leprosy patients, I always shake their hands and hug them, and at times I also touch the wounds formed from their disease. I do so because I possess correct knowledge about leprosy. My actions also convey a silent message to those who harbour a needless fear of leprosy: namely, that they should not fear someone with the disease.

Even so, on not a few occasions I am asked—by highly educated people, including government officials and people working in the media—whether it isn't true that leprosy is an incurable disease or a hereditary disease. On such occasions I am made indelibly aware of the deep-rooted prejudice that people still have toward leprosy—a realization that fills me with dismay.

After working in this area for many years, at some point I began to think that the history of human discrimination toward fellow human beings may have begun with leprosy. The world of course is home to numerous issues of serious discrimination that existed for long in the past and that today still give rise to tragedies: discrimination based on race, ethnic group or religion; discrimination based on gender, or social class, or occupation; discrimination based on physical features, and so on. René Girard (1923–2015), a social critic and expert in the anthropology of violence and religion, wrote about this in his *Des choses cachées depuis la fondation du monde* (English translation, *Things Hidden since the Foundation of the World*).

But when I ponder how the phenomenon of human discrimination arose within the history of the human race, and why it continues to flourish even now in the twenty-first century, I cannot help thinking that leprosy is at the heart of the matter, because societal reaction to this disease has consistently been ingrained with structures of exclusion and isolation. This holds true in all ages and regardless of country, ethnicity, religion or culture.

Since the dawn of history, leprosy has appeared in numerous written records the world over. Although opinion is divided as to whether such records in each instance refer precisely to leprosy, at the very least in the Bible, in both the Old and New Testaments, we find records of diseases believed to include leprosy. And according to those records, individuals who were found to have specific skin diseases were banished and isolated from their communities.

In Asia, the oldest record making mention of leprosy is said to be *Sushruta Samhita*, a compendium on diseases and their treatments written in India circa

600 BCE. It has been suggested, however, that even older references exist, including in a Chinese document from around 2500 BCE that records a disease thought to be leprosy.

From the Middle Ages onward, leprosy became rampant in Europe, creating social problems that demanded to be addressed. The response was to create facilities throughout the continent where leprosy patients would be confined. But being confined to such facilities effectively equated to being banished from society—a "death" sentence proclaimed to the living. Many such facilities were created at considerable distances from other human habitats—on the outskirts of villages or in distant fields—and their inmates were subjected to severe rules to ensure that their disease would not be passed on to others. In those days before effective treatments, it was believed the best way of preventing the disease from spreading any further was to isolate its patients.

Bettler und Gaukler, Dirnen und Henker (Beggars and Jesters, Whores and Hangmen), a work by Franz Irsigler and Arnold Lassotta, which focuses on people who were excluded from European society as communities became structured around cities in the Middle Ages, contains a passage about leprosy patients. It describes how persons with leprosy were treated in those days:

> When someone came down with the disease, serious consequences befell the person. By court ruling he was henceforth considered to be dead, and the severe responsibility of being isolated from the community of healthy people had to be carried out. In keeping with church formalities, he was blessed by the people of his parish like the dead ... including last rites and funeral rites. At the same time, he lost his fundamental personal rights ... in many aspects becoming treated as an incompetent ... and had to be incorporated into the community of the sick.

Even after the Middle Ages, the practice of isolating leprosy patients at locations far away from cities and villages continued to be implemented around the world. In those days long before globalization, times when transportation and communications were still largely lacking, the treatment accorded to leprosy patients alone was a common feature everywhere around the world.

In particular, numerous cases are found worldwide of remote islands used as isolation centres for leprosy patients. The list includes the Hawaiian island of Molokai, South Africa's Robben Island (widely known as the location where Nelson Mandela was imprisoned for twenty-seven years), Greece's Spinalonga and other islands in the Aegean, D'Arcy Island on Canada's west coast, Australia's Peel Island, Fiji's Makogai Island, Palau's "Leprosy Island", Culion Island in the Philippines, Korea's Sorok Island, Da Qin Island in China, and Malaysia's Jerejak Island. Four of Japan's national leprosariums—Nagashima Aiseien, Oshima Seishoen, Amami Wakoen and Miyako Nanseien—were also created on islands.

Even when they were not forcibly isolated, once a person was found to have leprosy he or she was inevitably expelled from the community. This occurred in all regions, all around the world, with the result that, having been ejected from their lands and stripped of any gainful employment, leprosy patients congregated and lived quiet lives in the shadows. In India, for example, even today there are more than 750 self-settled colonies that are home to people affected by leprosy and their families. These are communities founded by these individuals themselves, having nowhere else to go.

Normally, when a family member becomes seriously ill, whether a parent or a child, others in the family will lovingly nurse and take care of the stricken one. But in the case of leprosy, because discrimination is directed not only toward the patient but also toward his or her entire family, in many instances ties with the family are cut.

There have also been instances where patients have been isolated for their whole lives at special facilities and where, in order not to bring dishonour to their family or relatives, they have been compelled to adopt an alias. At the Gillis W. Long Hansen's Disease Center in Carville, Louisiana, for example—a national leprosarium—patients were not only forced to use aliases; they were also deprived of their right to vote. This situation continued into the 1940s.

These policies of isolation, which were established in an era when medical knowledge and treatment methods were both lacking, remained in place even after democratic principles took hold around the world and the concept of human rights became fully recognized. Leprosy patients were deprived of opportunities to be educated, to seek work or to marry; they were also forbidden to have their own families and to use their real names. Yet in spite of these egregious violations of their human rights, leprosy patients were also unable to raise their voices in protest against society. What they feared more than anything was to cause trouble for their families.

There were, of course, people whose hearts went out to leprosy patients and the distressing situation in which they were involuntarily placed, individuals who altruistically sought to help them in their plight. Father Damien de Veuster (1840–1889), of Belgian origin, dedicated his life to taking care of leprosy patients on Molokai, ultimately succumbing to the disease himself. In India, a country where leprosy was once rampant, Mahatma Gandhi (1869–1948) and Mother Teresa (1910–1997) expounded on the need to help those with the disease. Raoul Follereau (1903–1977), a French writer and journalist, appealed to the international community about leprosy issues and was responsible for inaugurating World Leprosy Day. Baba Amte (1914–2008), an Indian social worker and activist, founded communities where persons affected by leprosy could lead independent lives. They all raised their voices against the prejudices exhibited toward leprosy and strove to improve the situation of those it affected.

We must also not forget the many nameless people who have devoted themselves to the cause of those with leprosy. The names of such individuals are not carved in history, and perhaps their contributions lacked the force to resolve the underlying problems faced by people living with leprosy. But we should never allow ourselves to forget that there were hundreds of Father Damiens and hundreds of Mother Teresas who did everything within their power to support people who had been forsaken by their families and communities because of leprosy.

I believe that leprosy, in addition to being a medical issue, is the oldest continuing human rights issue in the history of mankind. As such, there is an imperative need to properly compile and pass on to future generations a history of the discrimination toward leprosy inflicted by mankind, and of the many people who have dedicated themselves to the cause of leprosy without fear of social prejudices. This historical backdrop I believe will make people look squarely at questions of overriding importance—why man discriminates against his fellow man, and why people infringe on the human rights of others—and will provide the impetus for thinking about these issues.

I also think that resolving the human rights issues surrounding leprosy could possibly serve as a rough guide, or model, for resolving a wide array of human rights issues that create tragic situations in countries across the globe. This is why I consider the resolution of human rights issues surrounding leprosy as both my most important endeavour and my life's work.

Japan's traditional view of leprosy: divine punishment

The existence of leprosy in Japan has been known, too, since antiquity. Although in more recent times the disease came to be called *rai* or *raibyō*, both renderings equivalent to "leprosy", originally the disease had no specific name and was referred to merely as *gōbyō*—literally, "karmic disease", a term that implies an illness inflicted on the sufferer as a consequence of his or her karma. Such a disease was viewed as a form of divine punishment.

One reason leprosy came to be viewed as divine punishment is said to derive from the Buddhist teaching to that effect, which steadily spread among

21

the Japanese public. The genesis of this thinking is partly responsible for incul-cating a strong sense of revulsion toward leprosy in the Japanese. *Gō*, i.e. karma, is a way of thought that sees events in life as the result of deeds—or, in this case more importantly, misdeeds—performed not only by the person but also by his or her parents, ancestors or incarnations in previous lives, consequences that get passed down to one's descendants even for generations. In this respect, all incurable diseases for which no effective treatments existed were considered *gōbyō*; but persons afflicted with leprosy in particular were said to bear the weight of especially dire karmas. The hideous physical defor-mities and disabilities wrought by leprosy were seen as forming the polar opposite to *Sukhāvatī*, the Pure Land of Bliss preached in Buddhism, which releases humans from all their sufferings; to have leprosy was tantamount to living in hell on earth. Clearly too, the more Buddhism put stress on the horrors of hell, the more people worshiped Buddha and prayed to be worthy of entry into Amitābha's Western Paradise.

From roughly the twelfth to the nineteenth centuries, the common revul-sion toward leprosy and the view that it was a disease of divine punishment found widespread expression in sutra-based ballads (*sekkyōbushi*) and musical narratives (*jōruri*). A factor contributing to the popularity of such tales was their characteristic inclusion of a pledge to the deities when making a vow: a pledge that stated, specifically, that "if I fail to keep my vow, I will willingly accept being inflicted with leprosy". To suffer the scourge of leprosy in life was in every way considered tantamount to dying and going to hell.

In the sixteenth century, Catholic missionaries who began arriving in Japan to proselytize also made efforts to help the country's leprosy patients. Their efforts were suspended in the early seventeenth century, however, when the shogunate government in Edo (Tokyo) passed edicts banning Christianity and launched suppressive campaigns against the religion. As a result, leprosy patients of those times had but two choices: driven from their homes and villages, to survive as itinerant beggars clustering at the entrances to Buddhist temples and Shinto shrines; or, to live at home in total seclusion, forever avoiding notice by others. This situation changed little even through the nine-teenth century, when Japan set out on the path to modernization.

In 1873, Gerhard Henrik Armauer Hansen (1841–1912) of Norway dis-covered that leprosy is an infectious disease caused by a rod-shaped bacillus, *Mycobacterium leprae*. Already by the end of the nineteenth century, research had brought to light the fact that leprosy is the outcome neither of "karma" nor of heredity. One can assume that this information reached Japan at the time as well, and yet the prejudice against this disease underwent no change.

On the contrary, attention came to focus anew on leprosy's aspect as an "infectious disease", and the fact that it passes from one person to another appears to have instilled excessive fear toward the disease on a scale even greater than before.

Even after the Meiji Restoration (1868), the movement that propelled Japan rapidly into the modernized world, people who came down with leprosy continued to abandon their homes, wander in the direst of straits, and cluster in isolated communities behind temples and shrines. Such communities, where they lived as mendicants, are said to have existed throughout the country.

The Leprosy Prevention Law of 1931 and "No Leprosy Patients in Our Prefecture" movement

Initiatives to help people with leprosy in modern-day Japan were started by two missionaries. Hannah Riddell (1855–1932) was an English missionary who arrived in Japan in 1891. She saw cases of leprosy for the first time during a cherry blossom-viewing excursion to Honmyoji, a temple in Kumamoto City known as the burial place of Kato Kiyomasa (1562–1611), a famed military commander of Japan's medieval period. Deeply touched by the pathetic plight of these mendicants, Riddell opened a temporary aid station close to the temple grounds. This facility later evolved into a hospital for leprosy patients: Kaishun Hospital (referred to in English as the Kumamoto Hospital of the Resurrection of Hope). Meanwhile, at roughly the same time, Father Germain-Léger Testevuide (1849–1891), a French missionary, founded a similar hospital—Koyama Fukusei Hospital—in Gotemba City, Shizuoka Prefecture. (Later, these facilities were given financial assistance by Empress Teimei, wife of Emperor Taisho.)

Japan in those times, while driving rapidly forward with its modernization ambitions, was also rushing quickly down the path to becoming a "first-class" power following its successive victories in the Sino-Japanese War of 1894–1895 and the Russo-Japanese War of 1904–1905. It was against this backdrop that the Act for Leprosy Prevention (Law No. 11) was promulgated on 18 March 1907.

The objective of this newly introduced legislation was to take itinerants suffering from leprosy and isolate and confine them at locations far away from heavily populated areas where others would see them. The Act further called for disinfection of the places where they had been, and for mandatory reporting. Following its promulgation, sanatoriums were progressively established at five locations around the archipelago, but in those days, when no effective

23

way of treating leprosy yet existed, in reality the newly created facilities were more in the nature of internment camps than sanatoriums. The Act for Leprosy Prevention was in truth passed only for national political motives: namely, to ensure that no persons with leprosy would be in a location where they might be noticed by foreign eyes, a "condition" deemed necessary for a country such as Japan that was aspiring to be a "first-class" nation.

Eventually, the Act for Leprosy Prevention was successively modified so that not just itinerant leprosy patients but all leprosy patients would be isolated and confined. These gradual changes then led to the establishment in 1931 of the Leprosy Prevention Law. Under the new law, all those with leprosy were to be totally isolated from Japanese society, meaning that patients who until then had voluntarily stayed confined to their homes so as to avoid notice, and even those whose symptoms were so mild as to constitute no impediment to living their daily lives, became targets for mandatory confinement.

The 1930s, when the Leprosy Prevention Law was enacted, was a decade when, commencing with the Mukden (or Manchurian) Incident of 1931, Japan began treading on a path leading to the Pacific War. All young males in the country were taught they had an essential duty to "serve their nation" by performing military service; but leprosy patients, their peripheral nerves in their limbs numbed from their disease, were unable to carry out that duty. As a consequence, patients were branded not only as "lepers" but also as citizens incapable of performing work for the nation, causing them to be socially ostracized all the more.

To compound matters, this period also saw the emergence of a clique of advocates of "eugenic cleansing": the conviction that in order for the Japanese race to maintain its superiority it was necessary to eliminate anyone of "inferior" endowments. And as prime examples of targets for such elimination, the eugenicists pointed to leprosy patients. Against this background there developed what came to be referred to as the "No Leprosy Patients in Our Prefecture" movement. The movement's aim was to ferret out any leprosy patients who had not been confined to a sanatorium and to place them in such institutions, down to the last man, woman and child. As the movement gathered momentum, prefectures throughout the country vied in seeking out all wayward leprosy patients within their territory. Clearly, the thinking underlying this action was the unquestioned belief that leprosy is an infectious and incurable disease, and therefore the most effective means of dealing with it is to isolate its patients permanently. As such, any person once diagnosed with leprosy should never, until the moment of death, be permitted to return to society. This notion came to be increasingly accepted as a given.

The daily lives of the patients who were crammed into the nation's sanatoriums as a result of this nationwide forced isolation policy were truly miserable. Sanatoriums everywhere were filled to overflowing, and all without sufficient numbers of doctors, nurses or staff to meet their needs. With no effective treatment provided to them, patients' disabilities became steadily more inhibiting. But owing to the egregious lack of human resources, those whose symptoms were relatively mild took care of their fellow patients who became immobile. Patients even had to produce their own food in order to survive, and not a few suffered exacerbation of their symptoms as a result of harsh labour. Many, unable to bear such lives, attempted to flee from their sanatorium. Those who were caught were punished by being placed in incarceration rooms on the sanatorium premises.

Leprosy patients were also compelled, largely without choice, to adopt an alias so as not to cause "trouble" for their families. Initially male and female inmates were housed separately within the sanatoriums, but when cases of pregnancy and childbirth occurred nonetheless, it became the general practice to abort all pregnancies and to force males to undergo a vasectomy. Astonishingly, such human rights violations continued for a remarkably long time—even in the postwar era as Japan underwent a rebirth as a democratic nation.

Leprosy becomes curable—but the isolation policy continues

In 1941 a chemotherapeutic drug, promin, was used for the first time on leprosy patients at the U.S. national leprosarium in Carville, Louisiana. Promin had originally been developed to treat tuberculosis, but clinical trials conducted at Carville revealed that it was effective against leprosy as well.

With Japan launching the war in the Pacific that same year, information concerning promin's breakthrough in the U.S. failed to reach Japan. Even in the midst of the war, however, there were Japanese researchers who devoted themselves to collecting information. The most prominent among them was Dr. Morizo Ishidate, who came to be known as the "father of chemotherapy in Japan". Dr. Ishidate served as first head of the pharmacology department at the University of Tokyo and later became the first chairman of the Board of Directors of the Sasakawa Memorial Health Foundation.

Dr. Ishidate learned of the drug promin's newfound effectiveness as a treatment against leprosy in a magazine he obtained via Switzerland, and he began an attempt to synthesize promin on his own. He succeeded, for the first time in Japan, in 1946, the year after the war ended. Dr. Ishidate next carried out trials at a sanatorium, with dramatic results. This seemingly miraculous event shed a bright ray of hope into the lives of the many patients of leprosy who had suffered for so long.

Hearing the news of promin's effectiveness, the nation's leprosy patients appealed to the Japanese government until finally, in 1949, the drug began to be administered to patients in large numbers.

As patients came to be treated with promin, the associations of leprosarium residents that had formed in the postwar years began actively demanding that patients who were cured by promin be allowed to leave their sanatorium. In response, the Ministry of Health and Welfare considered adding a provision for withdrawal from the nation's leprosariums to the standing Leprosy Prevention Law. In 1951 three directors of national leprosariums were called before a House of Councillors health and welfare committee. Contrary to expectations, however, the directors used the occasion to demand that the government instead impose even stricter forced isolation of leprosy patients, strengthen the powers vested in the sanatoriums, and institute regulations for punishments to be meted out to any patient who might flee from his or her place of confinement.

By 1951 five years had already passed since the promulgation of Japan's new constitution—a document that contained notions of respect for fundamental human rights. But the thinking of the nation's leprosy experts remained unchanged. There were exceptions: Noboru Ogasawara of Kyoto University, for example, who advocated an end to forced isolation and its replacement by outpatient treatment. But those who espoused opinions of this kind were still a small minority in those years.

The nation's leprosy patients, confronting the entrenched attitudes toward their plight, began, with a combination of deep anger and firm resolve, to speak up. In 1951 they formed a nationwide organization, the Japan Leprosy Association, and launched a movement calling for revision of the Leprosy Prevention Law of 1931, demanding that its provisions pertaining to forced confinement be deleted and its regulations on discipline and detention be abolished. The Association's demands notwithstanding, when a bill for revising the Leprosy Prevention Law was in due course submitted to the Diet, it failed to reflect those demands, and provisions tantamount to clear violations of human rights—forced isolation topping the list—were wholly retained. Leprosy patients protested violently using new tactics including hunger strikes and sit-ins.

Their protests aside, when the revised Leprosy Prevention Law was adopted in 1953, its provisions actually further strengthened the policy of isolation and confinement of all leprosy patients. At the same time, as with the original legislation of 1931, it contained no provisions allowing for cured patients to leave their sanatoriums.

The absence of a provision enabling a patient to leave the sanatorium after being cured of the illness was predicated on the premise that once a patient entered a facility, he or she should never be allowed to leave, even if cured. As the number of cured patients increased, clearly many would embrace the desire to leave the sanatorium and reintegrate into society; but so long as there was no provision in the Leprosy Prevention Law allowing for such withdrawals, the possibility of rejoining society remained beyond them. In this way the new Leprosy Prevention Law of 1953 was an anachronistic travesty.

For the sanatoriums, the need to continue obeying regulations of this kind on a permanent basis must have become untenable, for gradually cases emerged where, at the discretion of the sanatorium director, patients who had effectively been cured would be allowed to leave the premises on the pretext of taking a "long-term stay" outside the sanatorium. Additionally, regulations affecting passage outside the premises were gradually eased, and the sanatoriums themselves came to have gates with no guards on duty. Even so, many difficulties had to be overcome for any person affected by leprosy to achieve social reintegration.

To begin with, sanatorium inmates, even if they wished to return to their home towns, were in many instances totally estranged from the family members or relatives one might have expected to welcome them back. Jobs too were almost entirely elusive, there being almost no workplace willing to accept a "former leprosy patient". Social prejudice against leprosy was deep-rooted, and—as already noted—such prejudices were often based on groundless beliefs or images not at all in line with the true facts surrounding the disease. The nation's isolation policy, entrenched over many years, had set popular prejudice firmly in place.

The Leprosy Prevention Law of 1953 remained in effect until quite recently—1996, more than forty years after it was promulgated. The battle waged by leprosy patients against this law thus also continued for more than four decades. During this period Japan achieved postwar recovery; enjoyed an era of robust economic growth; became an economic powerhouse culminating in the widespread catchphrase of "Japan as Number One"; and then witnessed the bursting of its economic bubble and the start of a long period of recession referred to as the "lost decade" (or, more accurately, "lost decades"). Over the years, the vast majority of Japan's population forgot the

27

very existence of the Leprosy Prevention Law of 1953, as well as the existence of the many people who continued to suffer miserably because of this law. For people affected by leprosy, theirs was a lonely battle indeed.

Dr. Fujio Otani (1924–2010) was a physician who played a leading role in the struggle to have the Leprosy Prevention Law of 1953 rescinded. In his initial position in the employ of the Ministry of Health, for many years he devoted himself to improving the environment of the nation's leprosariums. Subsequently he served as chairman of a governmental Study Committee on Policy on Hansen's Disease Prevention, and later he became a member of the Board of Directors of the Sasakawa Memorial Health Foundation.

In 1997 Dr. Otani wrote the following in an article titled "Toward Realization of a 'Good Society': The True Significance of Abolishing the [Leprosy Prevention] Law" appearing in the newsletter of Tofu Kyokai, the Japanese Leprosy Foundation:

> The Leprosy Prevention Law of 1953 has been abolished—and yet there still remain a plethora of issues that we must reflect on and address in order to achieve a "good society". Why did it take so very long for the Leprosy Prevention Law, this grave wrongdoing, to be righted? Has the mechanism that enabled this misguided law to continue to exist for so long been elucidated? The prejudice and stigma suffered by patients and their families even today as a result of the extremely prolonged isolation are not easily erased, but how can we sweep them away and achieve a society free of prejudice? We must take up these issues, never relaxing our vigil now that the Leprosy Prevention Law itself has been abolished. We must seek after, and bring to full fruition, the true significance of the law's abolition.

In 1998, just two years after the Leprosy Prevention Law of 1953 was rescinded, 13 inmates of national sanatoriums in Kyushu—Kikuchi Keifuen in Kumamoto and Hoshizuka Keiaien in Kagoshima—initiated the first lawsuit in Japan against the government on the grounds of having suffered grave violation of their human rights as a result of the compulsory isolation policy that had long been in force.

In 2001 the Kumamoto District Court handed down its ruling in the case, finding the government responsible and awarding the plaintiffs 1.8 billion yen (approx. US$18 million). In response, the Ministry of Health, Labour and Welfare vigorously called for the court's ruling to be appealed; but the Prime Minister, Junichiro Koizumi, made the bold decision not to appeal, and that same year (2001) an amicable agreement was concluded between the government and the plaintiffs. These events had an impact on legal actions subsequently taken in Tokyo and Okayama, and ultimately the government agreed to compensate even persons affected by leprosy who had not taken part in the lawsuits. This was the first time a government had formally admitted that it had been at fault in isolating patients with leprosy.

Today, there are many young people in Japan who are altogether unaware that the disease of leprosy ever existed in this country. But the abolition of the Leprosy Prevention Law of 1953 and the lawsuits later filed, and won, against the Japanese government are events that occurred in the present era. As a Japanese, I feel that my fellow citizens and I must never forget that all of us, by virtue of a lack of understanding or lack of interest, played a role in the history of discrimination against our fellow human beings.

What Leprosy Elimination Efforts Have Already Achieved

Leprosy treatment developed rapidly in the 1940s

Through the aeons of human history, leprosy was long a disease for which no effective treatment existed. Prior to the early 1940s, one of the few treatments in use was chaulmoogra oil, oil extracted from the seeds of *Hydnocarpus wightianus*, a tree in the Achariaceae family, used in traditional Oriental medicine. Chaulmoogra oil was employed in various ways: ingested orally, applied topically to the skin, or administered intravenously. It has a very powerful odour, moreover, its effectiveness was anything but complete: at times its use triggered sensations of pain or discomfort. Physicians and patients relied on it nevertheless, having no alternative effective treatment to turn to.

This situation changed dramatically with confirmation in the 1930s of the effectiveness of sulfonamides—sulfa drugs—against bacterial infections. This was then followed by the development of a new drug, promin, or sodium glucosulfone, which demonstrated remarkable effectiveness in trials conducted on animals in 1941. Specifically promin, when administered to rats infected with rodent leprosy (*Mycobacterium lepraemurium*)—a disease closely resembling leprosy in humans—was shown to be highly effective.

The first trials of promin performed on humans took place at the Gillis W. Long Hansen's Disease Center in Carville, Louisiana. News concerning promin swiftly reached Japan, and, as noted earlier, Dr. Morizo Ishidate, then Professor Emeritus of the University of Tokyo, attempted to synthesize the drug despite the lack of sufficient materials caused by Japan's involvement in the Pacific War. He finally succeeded in his quest in 1946.

Promin was an ampule-type drug administered intravenously, but before long a new drug, dapsone, appeared that could be administered more easily, as it was taken orally. In the 1950s dapsone became the standard prescription drug to treat leprosy. But dapsone had to be taken continuously over many years, and eventually it became clear that over time *Mycobacterium leprae*, the leprosy bacillus, develops resistance to dapsone. Once this was known, an urgent search began for a treatment method to supersede dapsone.

Rising to this challenge was the newly founded Sasakawa Memorial Health Foundation (SMHF). Under the first chairman of the board, Dr. Morizo Ishidate, SMHF was very interested in scientific approaches to tackling leprosy problems. Its first international workshop was on the chemotherapy of leprosy, exploring alternatives to dapsone. Based on the workshop's recommendations, joint chemotherapy trials soon followed in South Korea, the Philippines and Thailand.

At around the same time, the WHO formed its own working group on leprosy therapy, and some of its members were involved in SMHF's joint chemotherapy trials. The results of these efforts by the WHO, SMHF and other agencies would eventually culminate in the recommendation by a WHO chemotherapy study group meeting in 1981 that multidrug therapy (MDT)—dapsone, clofazimine and rifampicin—be used as an alternative to dapsone monotherapy in treating for leprosy. In this way, in less than seven years after its inauguration, SMHF was able to make a contribution to advancing the treatment of leprosy.

Starting in 1982, treatment by MDT gradually came to be known around the world, and over the next three years its effectiveness in controlling leprosy also became widely recognized. Over the five-year period from 1986 to 1990, MDT drugs were distributed to roughly half the world. The treatment had an extremely high cure rate, and by using its three drugs in combination it was possible to suppress the generation of drug-resistant bacteria. MDT succeeded in having an impact on the treatment of leprosy not seen since the initial development of promin.

WHO sets elimination target

The WHO, seeing the effectiveness of MDT, took this development as a historic opportunity and decided to launch an aggressive and bold initiative relating to the treatment of leprosy. One manifestation of this initiative was the adoption of resolution WHA44.9 at the 44th World Health Assembly convened in May 1991. The resolution declared WHO's commitment "to attain the global elimination of leprosy as a public health problem by the year 2000". WHO also defined "elimination" as a prevalence rate below 1 case per 10,000 inhabitants.

LEARNING THE TRUTH ABOUT LEPROSY

Some people may think it odd to use the word "elimination" when a disease isn't totally eradicated, but the reason can be explained as follows. In the case of leprosy, it was felt at the time that if the prevalence rate could be brought down to below 1 case per 10,000, then this would be a low enough level for general health care services to cope with it and that a resurgence would be unlikely. In this sense "elimination" was to signify that leprosy was no longer a critical public health issue, while the setting of a numerical target was a way to mobilize resources and political commitment.

The individuals behind this were Dr. S.K. Noordeen (b. 1933), the director of the WHO's Action Programme for the Elimination of Leprosy, and Dr. Yo Yuasa (1926–2016), executive and medical director of the Sasakawa Memorial Health Foundation. From this time forward, conventional separately implemented measures for dealing with leprosy were superseded by a more integrated approach.

Another significant achievement in this connection was the development of "blister pack" packaging for pharmaceuticals. Blister packaging for leprosy drugs was conceived jointly by Dr. Yuasa and Dr. Hiroshi Nakajima (1928–2013), director of the WHO's Regional Office for the Western Pacific. Dr. Nakajima later also served as the WHO Director-General (1988–1998).

Conventionally, drugs had been passed by hand to patients wrapped in paper or newspaper. But with this method, which was used even with multiple drugs administered at the same time, patients often lost their medications or forgot to take them. Blister packs, in which individual doses of medicine are held in see-through plastic containers, eliminated these problems. Blister packs have the further advantage of maintaining the quality of their sealed drugs until they reach the hands of the patient, even in the world's most adverse environments.

Other factors that I believe influenced the WHO's setting of an elimination target include the development of solid support systems by NGOs and the like and the increased number of countries demonstrating strong interest in, and placing high priority on, the elimination of leprosy as a public health issue. In other words, besides the development of MDT treatment itself, the environment had become conducive to tackling leprosy.

When resolution WHA44.9 was passed back in 1991, leprosy was still a "public health issue" in 122 countries. Among them, India was thought to present a problem of especially large proportions.

India accounted for no less than two of every three new cases of leprosy found worldwide each year, and for that reason everyone concerned knew that in order for WHA44.9 to succeed, reducing the number of patients in

India would be essential. Given the challenges posed by India's size and diversity, however, surely no one at the time—when India's population was increasing explosively and had already exceeded 860 million—believed that leprosy could be eliminated there by the year 2000.

Still, nothing would be achievable unless a goal was set and steady ongoing efforts were made to attain it. At the same time, unless people firmly believed that the goal could be achieved and that they were capable of making accurate assessments of the situation, setting an elimination target would be meaningless.

What was important was to make the next move—a move that would take away people's doubts and feelings of uncertainty. This above all is what I kept in mind at the time.

Free distribution of drugs, worldwide

In 1994, the first International Conference on the Elimination of Leprosy as a Public Health Problem was convened in Hanoi, Vietnam. The foremost part of the agenda of the conference was to indicate more specific methods for achieving the target of eliminating leprosy by 2000.

The target had been set and everyone believed that setting it was both a correct and courageous act. And yet, no one at the time had a "strategy" for achieving it.

Against this backdrop, I decided to make a significant proposal at the Hanoi conference. I proposed that the Nippon Foundation would distribute, free of charge, MDT drugs worldwide for a period of five years starting in 1995. And I said the Nippon Foundation would provide US$50 million to the WHO to fund this programme.

The moment I announced my proposal, initially a great swell of excitement arose among the participants, followed by thunderous applause. From the stage I could clearly see the delegates talking to one another, with huge smiles on their faces. My offer was subsequently greeted with similar surprise and welcome by people involved in the leprosy issue all over the world.

Their reaction was altogether within reason, too, for the amount I had offered was the largest sum—by a wide margin—that the WHO had ever received from a private-sector source. The figure of US$50 million hadn't been decided on without basis, however. Our research had made us certain that a sum of this scale would be able to cover the cost, over five years, of the volume of MDT said to be necessary.

Carl von Clausewitz (1780–1831), the Prussian military strategist in the era of Napoleon Bonaparte, wrote in his book *On War* that there is no more important principle in war than never to divide or separate one's fighting strength. Similarly, the Chinese philosopher and military strategist Sun Tzu (fl. circa 500 BCE) wrote in his *Bingfa* (The Art of War) that a strategy should not be implemented in stages.

I too have always believed that in order to get something accomplished one should use all means available, never splitting up one's "strengths" unnecessarily. In this instance "strengths" consist not only of staff and cooperating parties but, at times, of close and equal relationships with heads of state and good relations with the mass media. A "budget"—funding—is obviously a component, too.

Through the mid-1970s the amount of money allocated by the WHO to fighting leprosy—approximately US$300,000 per year—was by no means adequate. The situation changed after 1974 when the Sasakawa Memorial Health Foundation offered to cooperate with financial assistance. Initially the amount of aid was of the order of US$1 million, but through the years it gradually increased, ultimately reaching US$14 million a year in 1995.

Dr. Halfdan Mahler, former Director-General of the WHO (1973–1988), once recalled, with a smile on his face, that the WHO's leprosy section had earlier been regarded as the organization's least vibrant section, but "thanks to Mr. Sasakawa it became the most vibrant".

Another important factor for driving things forward is to discover how to boost people's motivation.

Distributing MDT drugs free of charge also has ancillary benefits. As an example, when governments in developing countries suffering from fund shortages become free of the financial burden of purchasing MDT drugs, their budgets can be allocated to paying health workers and social workers to search out leprosy patients. In undeveloped lands, a great deal of effort is necessary in order to find patients among people who live far from villages or who live itinerant lives.

Governments may also be able to utilize their funds to conduct awareness programmes about leprosy treatment. NGOs that work to help leprosy patients too, once relieved of the burden of purchasing MDT drugs, can instead use their available budgets to fund such patient needs as plastic surgery treatment and prosthesis production. Also, for people operating at the grass-roots level, the knowledge that drugs effective against leprosy exist, and are available for free, provides them with a great boost.

I believed that these multifarious benefits would galvanize global initiatives to eliminate leprosy. And with this conviction in mind, I was confident that a sum of US$50 million would surely have meaning and impact beyond its face value.

Fortunately, after the first International Conference on the Elimination of Leprosy as a Public Health Problem, activities targeting leprosy elimination around the world became all the more robust. Free distribution of MDT drugs had great significance.

Travelling the world as the WHO Goodwill Ambassador

As the WHO's target date for the elimination of leprosy by 2000 approached, it became increasingly clear that while the goal would be achieved at the global level, the goal of reducing the prevalence rate to less than one case per 10,000 was unlikely to be achieved at a national level in a number of countries. The list of such countries included Angola, Brazil, the Central African Republic, the Democratic Republic of Congo, Guinea, Indonesia, Madagascar, Mozambique, Myanmar, Nepal and Niger. Bearing this in mind, it was decided to extend the target date. As to the question surrounding free distribution of MDT drugs beyond 2000, the Swiss pharmaceutical firm Novartis stepped forward with an offer to take over this initiative from the Nippon Foundation. As explained above, the free distribution of MDT drugs is crucial to the effort to eliminate leprosy, so Novartis has made a vital contribution in supplying MDT for free.

In 1999, the WHO formed the Global Alliance for the Elimination of Leprosy (GAEL) as a forum for strengthening cooperative ties among nations the world over. GAEL's first meeting on an international scale took place in New Delhi, India, in January 2001, and on that occasion a declaration was adopted—dubbed the Delhi Declaration—calling for the elimination of leprosy in all countries by 2005. It was at that meeting that I was appointed GAEL's Special Ambassador for the Elimination of Leprosy. In retrospect, this appointment was a turning point for me.

The first decision I made upon accepting the appointment was to become a "working ambassador". Some readers may think an ambassador doing work is altogether natural and in no way remarkable. But at many international institutions, being an "ambassador" is merely a title—and those ambassadors do no more than attend ceremonies and the like; they don't go out "into the field". This is something I—who am always determined to go directly into the field—have learned from personal experience.

Armed with my resolve to be a working ambassador, I determined to make it my job to actually walk through jungles and swamps, to penetrate into areas where leprosy is rampant, and to make direct contact with leprosy patients. More than aiming to carry out the duties of an ambassador, my intention was to use my title of Special Ambassador to achieve what normally can't be achieved.

I also made a point of personally going to see whether the MDT drugs were being properly delivered to health posts. As a result I ended up travelling all over the world, and from my travels I was able to confirm that MDT drugs are indeed reaching even patients in undeveloped areas with no electricity, no telephones, and no roads to speak of.

At the same time, I was also able to see with my own eyes and get to know the environments in which the people working in the front lines against leprosy must operate in some countries. Unless you see for yourself, it is not easy to grasp how different the situation is compared with that in a developed country.

To cite an example, at one health post in Africa the number of residents assigned to one person on duty can reach close to 5,000. Moreover, because those 5,000 people do not all live clustered in the same area, just visiting all of them is a task that entails great physical endurance. When I visited a village in northern Mozambique, I asked the woman at the health post to take me to a patient's home. "In that case, let's go next door," she said. But the place she then took me to was located more than a kilometre away.

In India, one general hospital typically serves approximately 1 million citizens, while the primary health centres subordinate to such hospitals normally see between 20,000 and 30,000 citizens. The sub-centres below the primary health centres are health posts serving some 5,000 citizens, but they have no doctors on duty whatsoever.

It is said that of the current world population of around 7 billion, roughly 2 billion people live in environments with limited or no access to modern medical health care. Nevertheless, I have often found MDT is getting through. No words of gratitude can suffice to thank all the people involved who make this possible.

Beyond the difficulties, hope appears

The campaign to eliminate leprosy subsequently continued on global scale. In 2001 the WHO was able to issue a formal declaration proclaiming that, on a global level, the target for eliminating leprosy—less than one case per population of 10,000—had been achieved.

But the WHO's declaration spoke to an achievement made on the grand scale of the entire world; individual countries, especially in the developing world, still faced many difficulties. I then realized that to reach the elimination target in the remaining nations, it would be important to visit countries in Asia and Africa where leprosy remained endemic and to offer advice and encouragement to their heads of state. I thus continued my activities in those respects, resolutely determined to eliminate the scourge of leprosy worldwide.

Regarding India in particular—the country said to hold the "key" to eliminating leprosy—I have paid up to seven visits a year, in total visiting the country altogether more than fifty times by now. On many occasions I have travelled to leprosy colonies in remote locations that even the local health workers may never been to.

In the light of my commitment to India, I was truly thrilled when, at the end of 2005, I learned that India had finally achieved the target of reducing the prevalence of leprosy to less than one case per 10,000 at the national level. Having been involved in India's fight against leprosy for so many years, I regarded this as a remarkable achievement on India's part, and I felt a huge sense of relief that this landmark had been reached.

The status of India notwithstanding, there still remained any number of countries that at the time were still unable to achieve "elimination" owing to political unrest stemming from armed conflicts, poverty, deep-rooted social stigma, and so on.

I visited those countries virtually every year, meeting with heads of state and asking for cooperation from local media. I am happy to note that after overcoming numerous challenges, countries such as Madagascar, the Democratic Republic of Congo, Angola, Mozambique and Nepal, where eliminating leprosy as a public health problem had seemed a far-off dream, were eventually able to achieve this public health milestone.

In 2018, there is only one country other than small island states where the elimination target has yet to be achieved, and that is Brazil.

I believe the history leading to the elimination of leprosy as a public health problem is a success story proving that humanity is capable of resolving its public health problems on a global scale. At the same time I also believe, very strongly, that this chronicle of international cooperation can become a role model for resolving many other international issues, among them religious and ethnic conflicts and discrimination.

Changing perceptions of leprosy

Through the years I have focused on three points necessary to realizing the elimination of leprosy: political commitment; media support; and cooperation among stakeholders.

Enlisting the cooperation of the media to report accurately on leprosy is an indispensable part of efforts to eliminate the disease and resolve the human rights issues associated with it.

One way I have sought to reach out to the media—and other social opinion-makers—is through publishing a newsletter in my capacity as the WHO Goodwill Ambassador for Leprosy Elimination. The newsletter covers leprosy from many different aspects and I hope that it has helped to familiarize people with a disease they may not have known much about, while disabusing them of mistaken notions they may have held. To date, over ninety issues have been published.

In a country the size of India, I felt a special strategy would be necessary, so I decided to host a series of media partnership workshops for journalists in different states, usually holding them in the state capitals, including Kolkata, Patna, Guwahati, Lucknow, Chennai, Jaipur, Ranchi and Pune. The aim was to encourage the spread of correct information about leprosy via local newspapers, TV and radio stations. Specifically, the workshops provided opportunities for the participants to consider how the media can contribute to restoring the dignity of persons affected by leprosy and eliminating all discrimination against them. We also urged the media participants to cease using the pejorative term "leper" and its equivalent in other languages, because of its dehumanizing implications, and to eschew reporting on leprosy in a sensational way. Besides local journalists, the workshops were also attended by a broad spectrum of participants—including the chief ministers of each state, health ministers, and members of government or NGOs involved in leprosy issues.

When the workshops were first launched, time and again we were astounded by the participants' general lack of knowledge concerning leprosy, and also by the grave misunderstanding of and prejudice directed toward the disease by representatives of local media.

In addition to being ignorant of the basic facts about the disease, they knew little or nothing of the lives of people forced to live in leprosy colonies because of society's prejudice against them. Even those who thought they knew something were sometimes mistaken in their belief that the disease was highly infectious or that it was hereditary.

That said, those who took part in the workshops approached them positively as an opportunity to learn about the disease—and to pass on what they had learned through articles and TV programmes. Today when I stack up the articles that appeared as a result of these workshops along with other articles that have been published about my leprosy activities in India over the years, they stand about 10 cm high.

But I do not wish to single out India's media for insensitive coverage of leprosy. Over the years I have lost count of the times it has come to my attention that papers and broadcasters in the West have blithely referred to people affected by leprosy as "lepers" when I feel they should know better. But in recent years I do see signs that media organizations are showing more understanding of the disease and the issues surrounding it, taking more care not to use discriminatory language, and I think this is a major step forward.

Persons affected by leprosy are the true protagonists

As chairman of the Nippon Foundation, I regularly press the point strongly to all staff members that just because we undertake humanitarian activities all around the world, we should never allow ourselves to become smug in thinking we are "doing good deeds" or "helping unfortunate people".

This is a teaching that I learned from my father, Ryoichi Sasakawa, and it is also an underlying precept of the Sasakawa Memorial Health Foundation founded by Professor Morizo Ishidate and Dr. Shigeaki Hinohara (1911–2017). The task we should be performing is "cooperation"—and this should never be confused with "assistance". Why? Because using the term "assistance" inevitably implies aiding persons affected by leprosy from a perspective of "providing alms from a lofty position". What we must never do is to force on them a passive attitude of accepting charity. The word "charity" has beautiful overtones, but we must keep in mind that at times its usage runs the risk of oppressing those who are its recipients.

As a constant reminder to ourselves, we must always keep in focus that our role consists of "cooperation"—the joining of forces for a common goal.

I also believe that the main protagonists in the fight against leprosy should be persons affected by leprosy themselves. Even after the disease is cured by MDT, discrimination—in the form of social ostracism—continues. What activities should those who live in such an environment pursue in order to restore their own human rights? This is something for the Nippon Foundation to think about in tandem with persons affected by leprosy as it plans its future activities.

Ultimately, it is for people affected by leprosy to declare: "We don't want another generation to experience the suffering we did." To overcome the deep-rooted misunderstandings and discrimination toward leprosy built up during the long course of history, truly persuasive powers are necessary—and only persons affected by leprosy, drawing on their personal stories, are capable of wielding them. This is something I have always been convinced of in my many years of working against leprosy.

Time and again I have borne witness to the fact that, more than my speaking hundreds of times on their behalf, one statement made directly by a person affected by leprosy is overwhelmingly persuasive. I appreciate that it takes great courage for someone who has been ostracized by society to speak out, but if the course of history is to be changed, such courage and self-confidence are needed.

More and more, courageous people affected by leprosy are speaking out, and over the years I have endeavoured to create opportunities for their voices to be heard at international meetings and in negotiations with government representatives.

One individual I have come to know and respect is Dr. P.K. Gopal. Dr. Gopal became the first chairman of the National Forum, a networking organization of residents of leprosy colonies across India launched in 2005 at my suggestion, with financial support from the Nippon Foundation.

Dr. Gopal came down with leprosy at the age of 12. The doctor who first examined him was unable to identify the cause of his symptoms, and it was only during his senior year at university that he learned that he had leprosy. As roughly ten years had passed since he contracted the disease, he was already suffering mild sensory paralysis, but after two years of treatment he was able to recover. Dr. Gopal received his doctoral degree for his dissertation on the social rehabilitation of persons affected by leprosy, a work he wrote based on his own personal experience as a caseworker. In 1986 he was presented a National Award from the President of India for his outstanding work in the rehabilitation of persons affected by leprosy.

Dr. Gopal has often stated that leprosy can truly be said to be cured only when all people affected by leprosy are able to live among society free of all discrimination. Yet he says that it wasn't so long ago that he himself failed to be accepted as an equal partner by experts involved in leprosy. Today he is highly respected for all he has done for persons affected by leprosy, and is a recipient of one of his country's highest civilian honours, the Padma Shri Award, presented to him in 2012.

It is not easy to surmount the fear stoked by prejudice and discrimination. Over the years, I have seen the courage it takes for a person affected by leprosy even to go to a hotel to attend a meeting of people involved in leprosy and converse with other participants over a cup of tea. In the south of India people affected by leprosy can sometimes be seen walking along holding a drinking cup made of metal. They are compelled to carry their own cup because when they order tea or water at a shop, the shop is loath to give them a cup to drink from. In India's West Bengal state, during a general election the locals once demanded that people affected by leprosy go to a separate polling station. Even today, some people worry whether they will be allowed into hotel or restaurant, or stay at a hotel.

With this in mind, it should be easy to understand what an epoch-making development it was for people who have long suffered social discrimination to create the National Forum, a networking organization through which they could address society for themselves.

In 2005, when the first meeting of the newly created National Forum drew to a close, a woman approached me from the audience with a big smile on her face. I will never forget what she said. "I arrived late and was unable to receive any mementos of the meeting, but today I received something I was never able to receive before in the forty years since I contracted leprosy: dignity as a human being."

The National Forum currently has representatives of persons affected by leprosy from more than twenty states, and a variety of activities are under way toward improving the lives of colony residents and restoring their dignity. I cooperated in and supported the National Forum's establishment and have continued to give my backing to the subsequent activities of its members. I was also instrumental in creating the Sasakawa-India Leprosy Foundation, with support from the Nippon Foundation, in 2007; it is dedicated to supporting people affected by leprosy in achieving social integration and economic independence.

A more detailed look at the work of the National Forum and the Sasakawa-India Leprosy Foundation can be found in Chapter 3.

Leprosy as a Human Rights Issue

Seeking support from the UN

The first time I spoke out about the human rights issues surrounding leprosy was at the Forum 2000 international conference convened in October 2001. Forum 2000 was initiated by Václav Havel (1936–2011), former Czech President, poet, playwright and global statesman who continuously fought for the cause of liberty. As the central figure in the "Velvet Revolution" that toppled communism in Czechoslovakia in 1989, Václav Havel served as President in the newly formed Czech Republic. Together with Elie Wiesel (1928–2016), writer, survivor of the Auschwitz concentration camp, and recipient of the Nobel Peace Prize, President Havel came up with the idea of establishing Forum 2000, a platform for global dialogue pursuing the path toward world peace, for the sake of the future of all humanity. They approached me with a request to join them in founding the forum, and in this way the three of us launched that grand project in 1997.

Forum 2000 was created as a vehicle for exchanges of opinion on issues of importance facing humanity in a globalizing world, and to make the results of these exchanges widely known to the general public. An annual event taking place in Prague, the Forum 2000 conferences through the years have brought together intellectual leaders, active worldwide, from a wide spectrum of backgrounds: political leaders, corporate leaders, prominent journalists, scholars, philosophers, writers, representatives of labour unions, NGOs and foundations, religious leaders, anti-establishment activists, and so on. The list of participants to date includes such diverse luminaries as Shimon Peres, Prince Hassan bin Talal, Bill Clinton, Henry Kissinger, Nelson Mandela, Mary Robinson, Sonia Gandhi, Oscar Arias Sánchez, Adam Michnik, Frederik Willem de Klerk, Hazel Henderson, José Ramos-Horta, Olusegun Obasanjo, Madeleine Albright, Francis Fukuyama, Peter Gabriel, Jeffrey Sachs, Archbishop Desmond Tutu, and His Holiness the 14th Dalai Lama. For many years, starting in 1997 and continuing through to 2011, the year President Havel died, I participated in the Forum 2000 conferences nearly every year, in part due to my role as one of its founders.

The main topic of the fifth Forum 2000 conference, in October 2001, was "Human Rights: Search for Global Responsibility". I delivered a keynote address titled "The Human Right to Health" in which I discussed leprosy from the human rights standpoint. My presentation appears to have had a powerful impact on the conference participants. To illustrate, after my speech Nobel Peace Prize laureate José Ramos-Horta, then Foreign Minister of Timor-Leste (East Timor), told me that until that moment he had been completely unaware of the existence of this crucial human rights issue in his country, and he vowed to investigate the matter immediately after returning home. I believe that Mr. Ramos-Horta was only one of many of the Forum's participants who came away with a new awareness of leprosy as a human rights issue.

Timor-Leste subsequently achieved elimination of leprosy as a public health problem in December 2010. A ceremony was held in March 2011 to celebrate this success, organized by Mr. Ramos-Horta in his new role as the country's President.

As an adjunct to the Forum 2000 programme, core participants created a mechanism known as the Shared Concern Initiative. Under this initiative, proclamations on various global issues faced by humanity were released through major global media. The proclamation issued in 2011 was, at my suggestion, on the topic of human rights and leprosy. I quote it here in full:

DISCRIMINATION AGAINST PEOPLE AFFECTED BY LEPROSY

Shared Concern Initiative Statement

February 2011

In December 2010, the UN General Assembly unanimously adopted a resolution approving principles and guidelines to end discrimination against persons affected by leprosy and their family members.

This resolution was the culmination of several years of lobbying of UN institutions by concerned stakeholders with the aim of focusing attention on an overlooked human rights issue: the social discrimination suffered by persons diagnosed with leprosy, which continues even after they are cured, and which also blights the lives of other family members.

For much of its long history, leprosy was feared as an incurable, disfiguring disease. People who came down with leprosy were ejected from their communities. They often ended up in isolated villages or remote islands, condemned by society to spend the rest of their days as social outcasts.

Today leprosy is cured by multidrug therapy (MDT), a course of treatment that kills 99.9 percent of the bacillus that causes leprosy after the first dose. Since MDT was introduced in the early 1980s, some 16 million people have been cured worldwide. Yet even after a person is free of the disease, they are not necessarily free of the discrimination. The stigma attached to leprosy has the potential to disrupt people's lives in ways that MDT alone cannot cure.

Educational opportunities, job prospects, married life, family relationships and community participation are all potentially threatened by leprosy. In some countries, discrimination is sanctioned by law, with leprosy grounds for divorce, for example. Even members of the medical profession have been known to discriminate against patients with leprosy.

Many of the problems faced by people affected by leprosy today stem from society's ignorance of the disease. It is mistakenly assumed to be highly contagious, and therefore sufferers are to be avoided at all costs. Moreover, deeply entrenched notions that the disease is divine punishment destroy the reputation and self-esteem of those thus diagnosed and cast a shadow over their families.

The principles and guidelines endorsed by the UN resolution go to the heart of the issues. They state that no one should be discriminated against on the grounds of having or having had leprosy. They call on governments to abolish discriminatory legislation and remove discriminatory language from official publications, provide the same range and quality of healthcare to persons affected by leprosy as to those with other diseases, and promote social inclusion.

LEARNING THE TRUTH ABOUT LEPROSY

But the resolution endorsing the principles and guidelines, although ultimately adopted by the United Nations General Assembly, is not a binding document. It can only recommend that states and civil society observe them. It is very important, therefore, that this resolution is not simply filed away and forgotten. It must be used by states as a roadmap to bring about an end to this unjust and intolerable discrimination.

We call on states to use the opportunity afforded by this historic resolution to work toward a society where people affected by leprosy and their family members can live with dignity and play their part in the life of the community. It is time to bring an end to this gross violation of human rights. Such a world is long overdue.

H.R.H. El Hassan bin Talal	*Prince of the Hashemite Kingdom of Jordan, President of the Club of Rome*
André Glucksmann	*Philosopher (France)*
Vartan Gregorian	*President of Carnegie Corporation (USA)*
Frederik Willem de Klerk	*Nobel Peace Prize laureate, former State President of South Africa*
Václav Havel	*Former President of the Czech Republic*
Michael Novak	*Religious philosopher (USA)*
Yohei Sasakawa	*Chairman of the Nippon Foundation, WHO Goodwill Ambassador for Leprosy Elimination*
Karel Schwarzenberg	*Minister of Foreign Affairs, Czech Republic*
Desmond Tutu	*Nobel Peace Prize laureate, Archbishop of Cape Town*
Grigory Yavlinsky	*Russian politician, leader of Yabloko Party*

Going back to the year 2001, after sensing that my address at Forum 2000 had aroused a vital response, I decided to take my initiative one step further. This time I would take up the issue of leprosy and human rights with the United Nations Commission on Human Rights (UNCHR). As is well known, health issues of global concern fall within the purview of the World Health Organization—which means that matters relating to leprosy as a medical issue are the concern of the WHO. But there are many other sides, besides the medical aspect, to leprosy, especially issues of stigma and discrimination. Many leprosy patients are unable to receive treatment for their disease because of their overarching fear of others finding out they have leprosy. Others remain closed off from their communities even after their physical ailment has been treated and cured. Issues such as these, I believed, lay outside the actual purview of the WHO's concerns, and that being the case, I mulled over the question of where to turn for leadership in treating leprosy as a human rights issue. The obvious answer was the United Nations.

The United Nations is the only institution where countries come together to consider and debate issues that affect the world as a whole. Yet to my great surprise, in the half-century since the UNCHR was founded, never—not even once—had the Commission taken up the topic of leprosy as a human rights issue. I was convinced, however, that this circumstance was owing—as in the case of the participants in Forum 2000—simply to a lack of awareness of its very existence. Somebody had to step forward and provide this information—correct information—and I felt that no one was more qualified to do this than those of us like myself who had been involved in leprosy issues for so many years.

The United Nations is a gathering spot for representatives of governments the world over. But what could I do at the UN to bring up the unrecognized human rights issues surrounding leprosy? At first I had no idea. And after all, I am merely a private citizen. At times like this, it's perhaps best to receive backup assistance from experts; but unfortunately at the time I also had no idea who would be the right people to approach as experts to discuss this matter and these issues with.

Ultimately I decided to take on the task, to bring up these matters at the UN, on my own. I knew full well that the task I was setting for myself would be fraught with extreme difficulties, as if trying to use a single nail to make a hole in a thick concrete wall. At first the nail would probably hit the wall and bounce right back at me. But I felt certain that if I kept hammering away over and over again, slowly but surely a hole would be opened in that wall. So long as I had a strong determination to continue without ever giving up, I would surely achieve the good results I was looking for. This is my conviction—something I learned from my many years of continuously fighting the battle against leprosy.

It was a thick wall, as expected

How then should I go about bringing up the issue of leprosy-related human rights with the UN? I didn't have a clue. What I decided to do first was to visit the Office of the United Nations High Commissioner for Human Rights in Geneva and make my appeal concerning the prejudice and discrimination surrounding the disease. The officer who met with me to hear my views on the occasion was Acting High Commissioner Dr. Bertrand Ramcharan. This was in July 2003.

I told Dr. Ramcharan that worldwide the number of victims of discrimination towards leprosy ran into the tens of millions, and I appealed for this matter to be understood as a human rights issue—and an issue that must somehow be addressed. After listening closely to what I said, Dr. Ramcharan offered me three pieces of advice. First, he recommended that I discuss the matter with Paul Hunt, who was then serving as UN Special Rapporteur on the right to the highest attainable standard of health. Second, he suggested that I hold a seminar for delegates attending the meeting of the UN Sub-Commission on the Promotion and Protection of Human Rights, which was scheduled for one month later. Third, he proposed that I hold a meeting at the UNOHCHR to discuss the issues I had raised with its staff members.

I immediately followed Dr. Ramcharan's advice and travelled to the UK to meet with Paul Hunt, professor at the University of Essex. On hearing my argument, Professor Hunt advised that I treat this matter within the parameters of "the right to the highest attainable standard of health". He did so because of what he said was the UNCHR's strong interest in issues of universal relevance: issues such as the human rights of women, of children, and of those in a state of poverty.

I had mild misgivings, however, toward treating leprosy-related human rights as a health issue. Deep down I felt that given the long history of negative treatment accorded to every aspect of leprosy, it should be treated as a category on its own—the human rights of leprosy—and not as just one of many diseases all lumped together.

With the kind intervention of Dr. Ramcharan, I next, as he had suggested, gave a presentation to the staff of the UNOHCHR. I prepared a mountain of materials of every kind for my talk, but in the end only five people attended. Quite frankly, I felt altogether discouraged, as if someone had taken the wind completely out of my sails. But I always keep in mind three things whenever I'm engaged in my global activities: to never let my passion slip away; to endure and be patient until the difficulty, no matter how large, is overcome; and to persevere until the desired result is achieved. A poorly attended presentation wasn't about to knock me down.

The only thing remaining was to hold a seminar for delegates to the meeting of the UN Sub-Commission on the Promotion and Protection of Human Rights. I had only a month to prepare, but I succeeded in holding a seminar in Geneva at the Palais des Nations, with presentations by persons affected by leprosy and representatives of NGOs. This was augmented by a display of photographs set out in the lobby. The individuals I invited to participate in the seminar were Dr. Arturo Cunanan of the Philippines, Birke Nigatu of Ethiopia, José Ramirez, Jr. of the U.S., his wife Magdalena Ramirez, and Dr. P.K. Gopal of India. Of these five, all but two (Mrs. Ramirez and

Dr. Cunanan, a physician at Culion Island whose grandfather was a leprosy patient) are persons affected by leprosy.

The schedule of events at the Sub-Commission's meeting was, as in the case of the UN General Assembly and other such gatherings, extremely tight, leaving the Sub-Commission members no time to attend a seminar like ours given by a collection of private citizens. To make matters more difficult, the rules in force at the Palais des Nations are extremely severe, including a pro-hibition on the distribution of pamphlets and the like. The only recourse we had under the circumstances was to try to attract the members' attention during their lunch break.

We came up with the idea of serving food and drinks right outside the room where we were holding the seminar, hoping the delegates would stop for a bite and listen to our reports as they ate. Two staff on hand from the Nippon Foundation—Satoshi Sugawara and Natsuko Tominaga—stopped the delegates as they emerged from the main conference hall for lunch, discreetly handed them our seminar pamphlet, and guided them toward our conference room.

These efforts aside, nearly all the delegates showed no interest and merely continued swiftly on their way out. Quite a few stopped and helped them-selves to the food we were offering, but only about ten or so actually pro-ceeded to come into the seminar room.

This demoralizing situation went on for several more years.

Taking the message to the UN

The first time I was given an opportunity to speak about leprosy as a human rights issue at the United Nations was in March 2004, at the 60th session of the UNCHR. I gave a speech before representatives of the 53 member states at the General Assembly, but I was allotted a mere three minutes. Somehow, in spite of the brevity of the time given to me, I had to make a strong impact on the delegates, arousing them to take an interest in the issue of leprosy and human rights.

I rehearsed my speech over and over, dozens of times, until finally I was able to read it in full within my allotted three minutes. But I was so absorbed in the task at hand that I didn't have the presence to measure how much of an impact, if any, I had made. It was only later that I found out that I was the very first person to ever speak formally at the UN on the issue of leprosy and discrimination.

Here is what I said on that occasion:

LEARNING THE TRUTH ABOUT LEPROSY

Mr. Chairperson, I am here to talk to you about leprosy and human rights. If left untreated, leprosy results in serious deformity. Therefore, through the ages, it has triggered fear and loathing. Patients have been isolated. Isolation led to discrimination. Discrimination turned people into pariahs.

Once affected, a person was fated to a lifetime more miserable than death.

Families were terrified of the shame if a member developed leprosy. They kept the leprosy-affected hidden from view. Or they simply abandoned them.

Today, leprosy is treatable. Since the early 1980s, 12 million people have been cured. 116 countries have seen the disease eliminated as a medical issue. Today, there are less than 600,000 known cases.

But, Mr. Chairperson, a problem remains. Discrimination is still rampant. Those cured of leprosy still can't marry. They can't get work. They can't go to school. They are still treated as outcasts. The problem is massive, global in scale.

Many still think leprosy is dangerous or hereditary. Many still see it as a divine punishment. And so millions live in isolation. They have no homes to return to. They are dead to their families.

As WHO goodwill ambassador for leprosy elimination, I spent 125 days last year travelling to 27 countries. I have seen this damage with my own eyes.

So Mr. Chairperson, why has this never been treated as a human rights issue? This is because these are abandoned people. They have had both their names and their identity stripped away. They cannot cry out for their rights. They are silenced people.

That is why I stand before you today. To draw your attention to these voiceless people.

Mr. Chairperson, leprosy is a human rights issue. I urge the members of this commission to rectify this problem. Develop a resolution. Support worldwide research. And create guidelines that guarantee freedom from discrimination for all affected by leprosy.

Thank you.

To augment my speech before the UNCHR General Assembly, we also organized a seminar on the sidelines at which persons affected by leprosy and others involved in leprosy issues from Brazil, the United States and India gave direct testimony of both the history and current state of discrimination in their respective countries. Professor Paul Hunt kindly agreed to be on the panel, along with WHO's health and human rights advisor, Helena Nygren-Krug.

The panel discussion drew an audience of only around ten people, but those who did attend listened closely to the words of Dr. Gopal, who spoke on behalf of persons affected by leprosy. He related how, until then, leprosy patients and persons affected by leprosy had never thought of the prejudicially induced discrimination inflicted upon them as a violation of their human rights, but rather only as their allotted fate—a fate they had simply resigned themselves to. But Dr. Gopal went on to proclaim his belief that, going forward, awareness would spread that eliminating leprosy-related discrimination is a social responsibility.

Several months after these events at the UN, in August 2004 we held a luncheon to which we invited the members of the UN's Sub-Commission on the Promotion and Protection of Human Rights. The event was realized through the cooperation of two individuals: Professor Yozo Yokota of Chuo University, who was a member of the Sub-Commission, and Professor Paulo Sérgio Pinheiro, who was then affiliated with the University of São Paulo. This was the first time I was afforded an opportunity to speak on the human rights issues surrounding leprosy directly to the Sub-Commission membership. Twenty-five of the twenty-six members attended.

The first person to speak up after hearing my remarks was Sub-Commission chairman Soli Sorabjee, a former Attorney General of India. He expressed his profound concern about the seriousness of leprosy issues in his own country, and he proposed that the Sub-Commission actively take up the issues surrounding leprosy. This commitment proposed by Mr. Sorabjee was of outstanding significance.

As a consequence of these proceedings, the UN Sub-Commission on the Promotion and Protection of Human Rights voted to formally take up the issue of discrimination toward leprosy patients, persons affected by leprosy, and their families. Thereupon Professor Yokota, who had long understood the significance of our activities and promised to provide us with his complete cooperation, was appointed Special Rapporteur tasked with conducting a fact-finding study on this issue.

The UN had finally been moved to take action.

Persons affected by leprosy speak before the UN

About six months after these new developments instituted at the United Nations, I next organized an international conference on leprosy as a human rights issue in Brazil. The event took place in Rio de Janeiro on 27 and 28 February 2005.

The conference had two objectives: to provide Professor Yokota and the other members of the Sub-Commission with an opportunity to hear the views of persons affected by leprosy directly, and to have them learn, at first hand, the situation of the social discrimination against leprosy by having them visit colony hospitals and other communities of people affected by the disease.

After this initial introduction in Brazil, Professor Yokota proceeded to carry out his duties as Special Rapporteur with further visits to India and South Africa, where he met with persons affected by leprosy and devoted himself to his mission with extreme diligence and dedication. His investigations culminated in May of the same year, 2005, with his introduction to the Sub-Commission of a motion calling for the elimination of discrimination against leprosy. In debating the matter, however, some members, in agreement with Professor Hunt, argued that this matter should be treated along with other diseases as a health-related human rights issue. In the face of such opposition, Professor Yokota and I both felt that reaching a consensus on dealing with leprosy as a human rights issue would be extremely difficult.

It was shortly thereafter, on 5 August 2005, while the issue was still being debated by the Sub-Commission, that I was given another opportunity to make an oral statement before its members. Again, the time I was allocated was a mere three minutes. Moreover, I was one of many NGO representatives on hand who had likewise been offered three minutes to make their various appeals to the membership. One after another, the representatives emerged from the back of the assembly hall and took their turn at the podium, making statements to the Sub-Commission's delegates, delivered with lightning speed. For any NGO, even just having spoken at the United Nations bestowed on the organization a coveted cachet, and this was why the format adopted by the UN was to give representatives a chance to express as much as humanly possible within three minutes—regardless of whether the Sub-Committee members, who were drawn from all over the world, were capable of understanding their content or not.

No one, I think, could possibly have seen this as the chance of a lifetime more than I did. But how, out of the enormous number of presentations being made—and most only halfheartedly—could I get the representatives to listen closely to my message? Gazing intently at the backs of the representatives, their ears fitted with earphones providing them with simultaneous translation, I felt strongly that, somehow, I had to make them turn and look my way.

Just as my turn was about to come, I suddenly hit upon an idea: to have the four persons affected by leprosy who had come with me into the assembly hall—from India, Ghana and Nepal—make statements. One of the four, Dr. Gopal, had been in situations such as this before, but the other three could never have imagined a day would come when they would find themselves in such a place as they were then in. For them, what I was about to ask came like a bolt out of the blue. "You're the lead actors today," I said suddenly. "I want you each to make a statement, thirty seconds long." Overcome with surprise and fear, they began shaking visibly.

Seconds later, the time had arrived. I stepped up to the microphone and began. "I would like to have statements made at this time by persons affected by leprosy," I said, whereupon the atmosphere in the hall changed completely. A stir immediately set in among the delegates, and as if in unison they all turned around in my direction. Some among them were eager to catch a glimpse of the faces of these "persons affected by leprosy" who were about to make their statements.

It was somewhat of a bizarre spectacle, a scene that I myself will never forget. But this is the reality of human rights surrounding leprosy, a reality that persons affected by leprosy confront every day.

The four of them were all magnificent. Partially in shock from the situation in which they suddenly found themselves, with a dignified air they proceeded to tell where they were from and what kind of discrimination they had experienced during their lives. A young woman affected by leprosy, Nevis Mary, spoke amid her tears of what it had been like for her growing up in India. All four of them ran over their allotted thirty seconds, but no one made any attempt to stop them. When they had finished, their faces overflowed with a sense of satisfaction. They each offered me words of their appreciation.

As I had intended—or rather thanks to the four individuals affected by leprosy who overcame their fear and nervousness and spoke so bravely before this intimidating audience—the outcome that day went well beyond what I had hoped for. This day proved to be what I consider a major step forward in the battle surrounding leprosy.

During the same session we invited the members of the Sub-Commission to dinner, where we showed them films depicting the harsh circumstances surrounding leprosy in India and Brazil. It was at this juncture that I felt the subject of leprosy as a human rights issue was, at long last, beginning to be understood.

It was after this that the Sub-Commission passed its second resolution. This time it went one step beyond the previous resolution and declared its resolve to eliminate discrimination against leprosy patients, persons affected by leprosy, and their families.

Appointment as Japanese Government Goodwill Ambassador for Leprosy

Just when I thought the stage had finally been set for a resolution on the issue to be passed by the United Nations Commission on Human Rights, a major obstacle suddenly appeared and blocked the way. In March 2006 the UNCHR underwent reorganization, being superseded by the new United Nations Human Rights Council (UNHRC); the Sub-Commission on the Promotion and Protection of Human Rights was simultaneously abolished. Immediately before it was disbanded, the Sub-Commission had passed a resolution calling for "continued deliberation within the UNHRC toward elimination of discrimination", but now the Sub-Commission members who had shown sympathy toward this issue were all scattered. To make matters worse, it was being said that under the new UNHRC, the authority of governmental representatives would be strengthened and the voice of NGOs like us would have less influence. I felt that we weren't just being thrust back to the starting block; we had been put at a new disadvantage, one or two steps behind the starting line. I had no intention of giving up, however, and with renewed determination I began urging the Japanese Foreign Ministry to take up this issue.

Luckily for us, even amid the reorganization from UNCHR to UNHRC, the stance shown by the Japanese Government held firm—with the result that "leprosy as a human rights issue" was placed second on the UNHRC's agenda (the first issue taken up was a Declaration of the Rights of Indigenous Peoples). In all, there were more than ten items on the UNHRC's agenda, and I believe the high priority accorded to this matter was attributable in large part to the power wielded by the Japanese Government.

The Japanese media, for reasons unknown, were almost entirely silent on these various events. Governments outside Japan and overseas NGOs, on the other hand, widely acknowledged the contribution made by the Japanese Government. I well understand that the media have an important role in monitoring how the government exercises its authority, but I would like to see it also inform the Japanese people of the wonderful work their government has done for the global community.

In 2007 the Japanese Government took the decision of making "appealing to the global community to eliminate discrimination against leprosy" a pillar of its diplomacy. It further took the step of designating me the Japanese Government Goodwill Ambassador for the Human Rights of Persons Affected by Leprosy who would play a central role in related initiatives. This appointment was a totally unexpected, happy surprise.

Shortly thereafter, Ambassador Ichiro Fujisaki of the Permanent Mission of Japan to the United Nations in Geneva (later Ambassador to the United States) began taking proactive steps on our behalf, once again urging the UNHRC to take up the issue of human rights surrounding leprosy at its plenary session. In this way a framework for our initiatives at the United Nations, which for a time was thought to have gone back to square one, was, with cooperation from the Japanese Ministry of Foreign Affairs, set in place of a kind never known earlier.

The Japanese Government went another step further and submitted a Resolution on Elimination of Discrimination against Persons Affected by Leprosy and their Family Members to the UNHRC.

In the twenty-first century, "human rights" has become a universally recognized concept within the entire global community. Today the world community does not countenance the existence of states that disregard human rights or establish regimes that oppress their citizens. And yet, the resolution of human rights issues is no simple matter—because human rights issues are always complexly intertwined with the interests and political positions of the parties concerned. This is why even issues involving clear human rights violations that grab the attention of the international community—discrimination against minorities, for example, or incarceration or mistreatment of political offenders—fail to make progress toward just resolutions. Even for an organization like the United Nations, coordinating the opposing interests or political positions of the countries or ethnic groups involved in such issues is difficult in the extreme.

Fortunately, leprosy is a topic that, compared with other human rights issues, is relatively immune to influences arising from conflicting interests. I had high hopes that many countries would support the resolution forwarded by the Japanese Government. But even with proposals of the utmost significance, getting them passed is impossible if political power relationships are misread, and therefore such possibilities must also be fully taken into consideration. This, like it or not, is the reality of the global community.

At that point I decided to call on the diplomatic missions of the twenty-seven principal member nations of the UNHRC to explain the aims of the resolution submitted by the Japanese Government and convince them of the need to adopt it. I went on this journey in the company of Akio Isomata, who was then serving as Minister at Japan's Permanent Mission to the United Nations and Other International Organizations in Geneva (now Minister and Deputy Head of Mission, Embassy of Japan in Canada).

Two countries especially stand out in my memories of this "pilgrimage": Cuba and China. It was said that because of political issues lurking in the background, both Cuba and China would oppose any proposal, of any kind, that was forwarded by the Japanese Government. It seemed like I might be wasting my time even going to those two countries, but I felt that without dialogue there could never be any understanding. So I went, first to Cuba's mission, where I met with the ambassador.

I opened the conversation in the following way. "I received a medal from the World Health Organization together with your great leader, Fidel Castro," I said. "I have great admiration for Mr. Castro. Recently, I also saw the film *The Motorcycle Diaries* about Mr. Castro's close comrade Che Guevara, and it moved me very much. As you know, Mr. Ambassador, Guevara, as a physician, took a great interest in leprosy. Seeing the film gave me the idea of comparing the leprosy issue to a motorcycle: with treatment of the disease as the front wheel and leprosy's human rights issues as the back wheel. There can be no resolution to the leprosy issue unless both wheels move forward in the same direction.

"Cuba is also extremely keen on issues concerning medical education, as illustrated by its acceptance of medical students from Timor-Leste," I continued. "And the reason medical care in Africa has advanced to where it is today, I firmly believe, is because of Cuba's efforts made to develop human resources. All of these undertakings are the product of Mr. Castro's leadership. And after all, the WHO's very creation owes a great deal to Mr. Castro's lofty input. The work I am doing today on behalf of leprosy is but an extension of the work instituted by Mr. Castro."

As I spoke with passion of my admiration for Mr. Castro, I noticed that tears were welling up in the Ambassador's eyes. The Ambassador then extended his hand to me. "As far as this matter you have brought up is concerned, I will take full responsibility for carrying it out," he smiled. "Don't worry about a thing, I assure you." It was a moment that drove home to me once again that if you approach someone with sincerity, your sentiments will surely resonate and yield a positive outcome.

My next target was China. The Chinese Ambassador was a man of few words, the type of person you could by no stretch of the imagination label as "affable". Here too, I began the conversation by relating how my father, Ryoichi Sasakawa, had met with Deng Xiaoping and how the two had found a great rapport between them. I then proceeded to the topic at hand.

"Sickness afflicts everyone," I began, "regardless of political persuasion, ideology or religion. It's an affliction common to all humankind, crossing all national borders. If you agree on this point, then I ask you, please, to cooperate with us in this matter."

The Chinese Ambassador showed none of the deep emotion expressed by his Cuban counterpart, but he immediately pledged that he would contact his superiors back home and offer us his country's cooperation.

As I have thought all along, you cannot judge someone until you have personally met them and talked with them. And if you approach them with conviction, even things that hypothetically would appear to be impossible invariably become possible. Akio Isomata, who accompanied me on both of these visits, was left speechless at the way I had secured the cooperation, on the spot, of both the Cuban and Chinese ambassadors, but this was but another of the many lessons I had been taught by my father.

The world's first resolution, unanimously adopted, to end discrimination against leprosy

Although not a very familiar notion in Japan, in the West the authority wielded by a judge in a court of law, or by the person in charge of proceedings in a formal setting, when he or she pounds the gavel, is absolute. Once a decision has been declared, accompanied by the sound of the gavel, no one, no matter who it might be, can voice an objection. The door to debate on the matter has been closed, and everyone involved is obliged to strictly comply with the decision or statement that has been rendered.

On 18 June 2008, at the 8th regular session of the United Nations Human Rights Council held at the Palais des Nations in Geneva, a motion, drawn up by the Japanese Government and jointly forwarded by fifty-nine member nations, was taken up calling for the "elimination of discrimination against persons affected by leprosy and their family members". The Council chairman addressed the participants with a proposal that the motion be adopted by consensus, without voting, and he asked if anyone had any objection to his suggestion. No nation voiced an objection—and thus the motion was unanimously approved and adopted. When the chairman's gavel sounded, it marked an event of truly historic significance.

Among the fifty-nine nations that jointly submitted this epoch-making motion were Cuba and China, the two nations that had been said to oppose any proposal that might be made by the Government of Japan. True, the ambassadors of both countries had given me their pledge to cooperate, which I had taken as their agreement to vote in favour of the resolution when taken up for consideration. But in the end both Cuba and China had added their names to the list of countries that submitted the motion itself.

I was told that the passage of this leprosy resolution also marked a rare occasion in history when the world had fully united on an issue concerning human rights—something that, no matter what the specifics might entail, was said to be inevitably greeted by a vote of opposition from somewhere.

Even resolutions relating to HIV and AIDS had met with opposition from certain quarters.

The motion passed at the UNHRC session also called for the preparation of principles and guidelines for eliminating discrimination against persons affected by leprosy. A request to this effect was issued to the UNHRC's Advisory Committee, and committee member Shigeki Sakamoto, then Professor of International Law at Kobe University, was appointed to draw up what came to be formally referred to as the "Principles and Guidelines".

In January 2009 the Office of the United Nations High Commissioner for Human Rights called a meeting to discuss how to cooperate with Professor Sakamoto in collecting and exchanging information. Professor Sakamoto's proposed principles and guidelines were then taken up for consideration at an Advisory Committee meeting convened that August.

It was here that a problem reared its head again. Miguel Alfonso Martinez, the Cuban representative, issued a strong appeal for the need to isolate leprosy patients, even temporarily, from the standpoint of public health in view of the communicable nature, he claimed, of this disease. As a result of Mr. Martinez's advocacy, the final version of the proposed "Principles and Guidelines" retained wording suggestive of the potential for temporary isolation.

We vehemently opposed the inclusion of the word "isolation" on the grounds that it, more than anything else, symbolized discrimination against leprosy. Equally strong opposition was voiced by a number of international NGOs, among them members of the International Federation of Anti-Leprosy Associations, such as Netherlands Leprosy Relief. Professor Sakamoto and others involved in preparing the principles and guidelines responded to this challenge, pooling their collective wisdom to hammer out a solution to the matter. In the end, the word "isolation" was eliminated from the final draft.

In August 2010 the Chilean representative on the Advisory Committee, José Antonio Bengoa Cabello, strongly advocated that a clause be included clearly stating that existing facilities where persons affected by leprosy and their family members had previously been forcibly interned be progressively phased out. In response, we argued that including such a clause could potentially infringe on the rights of persons who desired to continue living in such facilities, and we succeeded in reaching a unanimous opinion not to add this provision.

Finally, in September 2010, after a series of twists and turns in the preparation of its exact content and wording by the Advisory Committee, the resolution on the elimination of discrimination against persons affected by leprosy and their family members, including the "Principles and Guidelines", was unanimously adopted at the fifteenth regular session of the UNHRC.

With matters set in motion, at this juncture I called on the Japanese Ministry of Foreign Affairs to submit a resolution to the UN General Assembly in New York. With the full backing of the Permanent Mission of Japan to the United Nations, including head of the Foreign Ministry's Human Rights and Humanitarian Affairs Division, Mitsuko Shino, on 21 December 2010 the resolution proposed by the Government of Japan, calling for the elimination of discrimination against persons affected by leprosy and their families and the adoption of the "Principles and Guidelines", was unanimously passed by the 192 member nations of the UN. No fewer than eighty-four countries had joined together in submitting this proposal.

Here, I would like to introduce the complete text of the "Principles":

1. Persons affected by leprosy and their family members should be treated as people with dignity and are entitled, on an equal basis with others, to all the human rights and fundamental freedoms proclaimed in the Universal Declaration of Human Rights, as well as in other relevant international human rights instruments to which their respective States are parties, including the International Covenant on Economic, Social and Cultural Rights, the International Covenant on Civil and Political Rights, and the Convention on the Rights of Persons with Disabilities.
2. Persons affected by leprosy and their family members should not be discriminated against on the grounds of having or having had leprosy.
3. Persons affected by leprosy and their family members should have the same rights as everyone else with respect to marriage, family and parenthood. To this end:
    (a) No one should be denied the right to marry on the grounds of leprosy;
    (b) Leprosy should not constitute a ground for divorce;
    (c) A child should not be separated from his or her parents on the grounds of leprosy.
4. Persons affected by leprosy and their family members should have the same rights as everyone else in relation to full citizenship and obtaining identity documents.
5. Persons affected by leprosy and their family members should have the right to serve the public, on an equal basis with others, including the right to stand for elections and to hold office at all levels of government.
6. Persons affected by leprosy and their family members should have the right to work in an environment that is inclusive and to be treated on an equal basis with others in all policies and processes related to recruit-

ment, hiring, promotion, salary, continuance of employment and career advancement.

7. Persons affected by leprosy and their family members should not be denied admission to or be expelled from schools or training programmes on the grounds of leprosy.
8. Persons affected by leprosy and their family members are entitled to develop their human potential to the fullest extent, and to fully realize their dignity and self-worth. Persons affected by leprosy and their family members who have been empowered and who have had the opportunity to develop their abilities can be powerful agents of social change.
9. Persons affected by leprosy and their family members have the right to be, and should be, actively involved in decision-making processes regarding policies and programmes that directly concern their lives.

Taking the Principles and Guidelines to the world

The unanimous adoption of these principles by the UN General Assembly was a momentous event. It took place seven and a half years after I had first knocked on the UNCHR's door in 2003, a complete novice at what I was seeking to accomplish.

Even with this achievement, my battle was not at an end. Needless to say, the adoption of resolutions by the UNHRC and the UN General Assembly did not translate into the immediate elimination of the stigma associated with and discrimination demonstrated toward persons affected by leprosy and their family members.

To ensure that this hard-won UN resolution and its accompanying "Principles and Guidelines" would not exist in name only, I devised two tactics. The first was to hold a series of regional symposiums in the Americas, Asia, Africa, the Middle East and Europe on leprosy and human rights. The second was to form an International Working Group to look into ways of implementing the principles and guidelines.

The first symposium was held in Rio de Janeiro, Brazil, in January 2012. The symposium was attended by numerous representatives of human rights organizations and international NGOs, UN affiliates, and leprosy patients and people affected by leprosy. It was at this symposium that a resolution was adopted to form the International Working Group.

The second symposium took place in Delhi, India, in October 2012. Among the participants on that occasion were the chairman of India's National Human Rights Commission (NHRC) and several members of the

Indian Parliament, and a highlight was their announcement of the formation of a cross-party forum tasked with combating leprosy. The third symposium was held in Ethiopia, attended by that country's Prime Minister, Hailemariam Desalegn. It provided a crucial opportunity to make an appeal concerning leprosy and human rights to all the member nations of the African Union. As at the symposium in India, where many people affected by leprosy had participated in response to a call issued by the National Forum, in Ethiopia too more than a hundred persons affected took part in response to a call by ENAPAL, the Ethiopian National Association of Persons Affected by Leprosy.

Rabat, the capital of Morocco, was the site of the fourth symposium. The event was held with the full cooperation of the Moroccan Government. Participating on behalf of that country's people affected by leprosy was Naima Azzouzi. Ms. Azzouzi had been diagnosed with leprosy at the age of nine and placed in a facility where she remained shut off from outside contact. She spoke of the newly formed association of people affected by leprosy in her country, Morocco's first such organization, in which she was serving as president.

The fifth and final international symposium took place in Geneva in 2015. Here too, a remarkable number of people affected by leprosy participated, including individuals from Brazil, China, Colombia, Ethiopia, Ghana, India, Indonesia, Morocco and the Philippines. It was at this final symposium that the IWG took the opportunity to report on its activities.

Two individuals played central roles in the organization: Professor Yozo Yokota of Chuo University, who had made selfless efforts as a former member of the UN Sub-Commission on the Promotion and Protection of Human Rights; and Professor Shigeki Sakamoto of Kobe University, who had drafted the "Principles and Guidelines". Its members also included human rights experts from around the world and persons affected by leprosy.

The IWG had two overriding tasks: to devise measures for protecting people affected by leprosy, as well as their family members, from discrimination and discriminatory treatment; and to draft an action plan for achieving broad social recognition and realization of the "Principles and Guidelines". In all, the IWG met on four occasions: in October 2012, March 2013, August 2013, and October 2014.

The results of the IWG's investigations and deliberations, which they relayed to the symposium in Geneva, were subsequently compiled into a final report that was submitted to the UN. The report recommended that addressing leprosy-related issues should be a responsibility at the national level, with all discriminatory laws and customs abolished. In every country, it advocated, government agencies at both the national and local levels—judiciary, legislature and executive—should act in accordance with the Principles and Guidelines, and an action plan matched to the situation of each particular country should be drawn up and implemented. In addition, the report urged strongly that the principal roles in these matters should be played by people affected by leprosy themselves.

The report also pushed for religious leaders of all persuasions to take a role in fighting leprosy-related discrimination. One demand made of religious leaders was to teach their followers not to use the word "leper". As will be discussed below, this entreaty bore fruit at an international symposium subsequently held at the Vatican.

Among the recommendations issued by the IWG, especially important was its suggestion as to how these issues should be dealt with going forward. The report called on the UNHRC Advisory Committee to prepare, at the international level, the necessary follow-up mechanisms. In response to this call, under a proposal drafted by the Japanese Government, in 2015 the UNHRC unanimously adopted a resolution requesting the Advisory Committee to undertake a study reviewing the implementation of the Principles and Guidelines, together with any obstacles to their implementation, and submit a report. Accordingly, Mr. Imeru Yigezu of Ethiopia, a member of the Advisory Committee, was chosen to be a rapporteur for the drafting committee. Over a period of two years, he was charged with examining the progress made in eliminating discrimination in countries around the world, and reporting back with recommendations for achieving further progress in future.

After two years of investigation, the report submitted by Mr. Yigezu stressed that in order to put the Principles and Guidelines into practice, it was necessary to establish mechanisms including a special mandate for follow-up, monitoring and reporting within the UNHRC itself.

After Mr. Yigezu's report was submitted to the UNHRC in June 2017, the Japanese Government moved at full speed to secure backers. Without delay a formal proposal was made to appoint a Special Rapporteur.

To be honest, I hadn't expected the UNHRC to move so quickly toward appointing a Special Rapporteur, and the speed with which events developed was owing entirely to the strong commitment and magnificent diplomatic efforts of everyone at the Permanent Mission of Japan (to the United Nations and Other International Organizations) in Geneva. Special mention must be made of Mitsuko Shino, who in 2008, in her position at the time of director of the Japanese Ministry of Foreign Affairs' Human Rights and Humanitarian Affairs Division, had contributed greatly to the adoption of the UN resolution. After serving for several years as Japan's Ambassador to Iceland, Ms. Shino had become Ambassador of the Human Rights and Humanitarian Affairs Division in Geneva, and thanks to her extraordinary diplomatic skills and selfless dedication to promotion of her cause, a joint proposal backed by 43 countries—including Brazil, Ethiopia, Vietnam, Ghana and Egypt—was submitted.

These efforts paid off, and the resolution jointly proposed by 43 countries was unanimously passed at the 35th session of the UNHRC, paving the way for the appointment of a Special Rapporteur on leprosy-related issues.

In September 2017 the UNHRC approved the appointment of Dr. Alice Cruz of Portugal for a three-year term. A medical anthropologist, Ms. Cruz has experience as a volunteer working with the Brazilian non-governmental organization MORHAN (Movement for the Reintegration of Persons Affected by Hansen's Disease), and is well versed in leprosy issues. I was thrilled at her appointment and look forward to what will be achieved during her term.

Shining a spotlight through the Global Appeal

To promote the human rights of all persons affected by leprosy all around the world, I launched—and remain proactively involved in—an initiative known as the Global Appeal. The annual appeal draws attention to the barriers that persons affected by leprosy and their family members face and is endorsed by a different set of influential individuals and organizations each year who lend their voices to the call for a world free of leprosy and the discrimination it causes. The first Global Appeal was held in New Delhi, India, on 29 January 2006, and since then a corresponding event has been carried out every year on or near World Leprosy Day, which falls on the last Sunday of January.

Signatories of the first Global Appeal included five Nobel Peace Prize laureates: former U.S. President Jimmy Carter, former President of Costa Rica Oscar Arias, His Holiness the 14th Dalai Lama, Archbishop Emeritus of Cape Town Desmond Tutu, and Elie Wiesel, President of the Elie Wiesel Foundation for Humanity. Other dignitaries who took part were Prince of the Jordanian Hashemite Royal Dynasty el-Hassan bin Talal, President of the Czech Republic Václav Havel, President Luiz Inácio Lula da Silva of the Federative Republic of Brazil, President Olusegun Obasanjo of the Federal Republic of Nigeria, former United Nations High Commissioner for Human Rights Mary Robinson, and former President R. Venkataraman of India. The total number of signatories, myself included, was twelve.

The Global Appeal of 2006 "call[ed] on people all over the world to change their perception and foster an environment in which leprosy patients, cured persons and their families can lead normal lives free from stigma and discrimination". It also "urge[d] governments themselves to seriously consider this issue and act to improve the present situation with a sense of urgency", and further "appeal[ed] to the UN Commission on Human Rights to take up this matter as an item on its agenda, and request[ed] that it issue principles and guidelines for governments to follow in eliminating all discrimination against people affected by leprosy".

At the time, in January 2006, I was still in the throes of rushing about in my quest to have this issue addressed within the framework of the United Nations. The day after this first Global Appeal was released in New Delhi, the Government of India issued a formal statement announcing the elimination of leprosy as a public health problem. It was a timely turn of events.

The second Global Appeal, in January 2007, was issued in Manila, the Philippines, its signatories consisting of representatives of persons affected by leprosy from sixteen different countries. The third Global Appeal was launched in 2008 from the Royal Society of Medicine in London, attended by representatives of prominent NGOs working for human rights issues, including Amnesty International and International Save the Children Alliance, among others. In 2009, the fourth Global Appeal, announced at Church House, adjacent to Westminster Abbey in London, brought together representatives of the world's major religions, including Christianity, Islam, Buddhism, Russian Orthodox Christianity and Hinduism. In 2010, the venue shifted to Mumbai, India, and that year's Global Appeal was signed by top executives of some of the world's leading business corporations, including Toyota Motor Corporation, Virgin Group, Tata Group, Mahindra Group, Johnson & Johnson, and Renault.

In 2011, the Global Appeal launch took place at Peking University, and the signatories consisted of the heads of more than a hundred of the world's leading universities. In 2012, with endorsement from the Geneva-based World Medical Association, members of the medical profession participated as the Global Appeal venue moved to São Paulo, Brazil. In 2013, the venue returned to London—this hosted by the Law Society—endorsed by the International Bar Association and forty-six member associations from forty countries and one region. Global Appeal 2014 shifted to Jakarta, Indonesia, with national human rights institutions from thirty-nine countries and regions providing their valuable endorsement. In 2015, the appeal was supported by the International Council of Nurses, in 2016 by Junior Chamber International and its branches in 130 countries, in 2017 by the Inter-Parliamentary Union and its 173 member parliaments and eleven associate members, and in 2018 by Disabled Peoples' International representing ninety-one national organizations and assemblies.

The discrimination targeted at leprosy patients, persons affected by leprosy and their family members extends into a variety of areas including profession, gender, education and community life. As such, by winning endorsement from influential leaders, people in socially important positions, in various spheres—NGOs, religion, the corporate sector, education and law, among others—and issuing joint messages calling for the elimination of such discrimination, we have drawn the attention of people all over the world, stressing the importance of addressing leprosy as a human rights issue.

I am committed to continuing the Global Appeal initiative for as long as is necessary—until the day comes when discrimination against leprosy has disappeared from the world. When, I wonder, might that day come?

2

RYOICHI SASAKAWA AND THE NIPPON FOUNDATION

Motorboat Racing and Humanitarian Activities

Discrimination inflicted on Ryoichi Sasakawa

Ryoichi Sasakawa, my father, is widely known outside Japan as a globally active philanthropist who during his lifetime contributed, among other achievements, to the elimination of smallpox—there is even a bust of him inside the headquarters of the World Health Organization in Geneva; but within Japan, for some reason, he suffers an unsavoury reputation. The domestic media have long depicted him in an unfavourable light: as a right-wing heavyweight in the years before World War II, as an accused war criminal locked up in Sugamo Prison after the war, and as a freewheeling manipulator of the proceeds from Japan's motorboat racing industry in the years after the country staged its remarkable recovery. "A behind-the-scenes fixer" is a description commonly used by the media to define him. I have always found this blatant contrast between my father's positive reputation abroad and his negative repute at home quite odd. After all, he was but one human being; he did not lead two separate lives.

In pre-war years my father led a group known as the Kokusui Taishū-tō (occasionally rendered in English as the Patriotic People's Party, or PPP), and there is no denying the fact that he was a nationalistic political activist who vociferously preached the virtues of self-sacrifice for the sake of one's country. In view of his political stirrings and the disturbances caused by his followers, it is easy to imagine why in the public's eye my father came to be regarded as a purveyor of dangerous ideas. And yet today, thanks to studies by historians and political scientists, my father's reputation is gradually being rehabilitated, his words and deeds no longer judged as having been exclusively rooted in right-wing dogma or ultra-nationalist beliefs.

The principle my father held most sacrosanct in the pre-war years was standing up for the masses, never truckling to those in positions of power. The ideals espoused by him in those years are perhaps nowhere more succinctly summarized than in the following passage from a 2011 biography written by Takashi Ito (b. 1932), one of the foremost authorities on Japan's contemporary political history:

> Sasakawa often attacked the wealthy, leaders of the powerful industrial conglomerates (*zaibatsu*), businessmen with strong political ties, politicians, corrupt civil servants and heartless men of authority, always describing himself as a representative of the masses, the hoi polloi. He consistently and repeatedly asserted that he played a "non-central" role in the philosophy he embraced, that his commitment was to the "public" without regard for his own personal interests. This was a manifestation of the self-discipline that he maintained throughout his life.

If one were to sum up my father's policy accurately in one word, I believe that word should be "patriotism"—not "nationalism" or "ultra-nationalism" as those of a narrow viewpoint have at times suggested. My father loved the country of his birth, he grieved over Japan's present and future, and, on behalf of the masses who embraced those same sentiments, he was not afraid to speak up to heartless men in positions of authority.

In order to bring this policy of his to fruition, in 1942, while the nation was embroiled in war at its height, my father ran for election to the Imperial Diet as a member of the House of Representatives—and won. During his election campaign he proclaimed that he was prepared to serve as a "clearing house" always ready to take on any and all discontent or disgruntlement his fellow countrymen might have, and he pledged to work on the people's behalf. Once in the Diet, he voiced strong outright opposition to the election process conducted under the Imperial Rule Assistance Association's authority, and he also appealed for improvement in how inmates incarcerated in the nation's prisons were being treated and in how prosecutors and the police were performing their duties. In those wartime days, my father was the only Diet member who was bold enough to voice views of these kinds.

After the war, my father was marked as a Class A war criminal and sent to Sugamo Prison, but no clear reason for branding him this way is in evidence. In the first place, when Japan was at war my father stood firmly on the side of the common people as a member of the Diet—but as a member of the opposition camp, not the party in power, so he was not in any position of importance of the kind that might warrant description as a war criminal. If a feasible cause does exist, the only possibility is the fact that on more than twenty occasions my father held public meetings at which he spoke critically of GHQ, the headquarters overseeing the occupation of Japan, and these speeches could potentially have been viewed as "anti-American activities". In the end, my father spent three years in detention at Sugamo, only to be eventually released without having been formally indicted.

During his period of detention my father kept a highly detailed diary, and also wrote an enormous number of letters addressed to family members and to others he felt it necessary to contact. Together these documents provide a vivid record of his interactions with the suspected war criminals similarly detained at Sugamo—the men who had led the country during the wartime period—and of the personalities of those individuals. He also sent numerous letters addressed to President Harry Truman and General Douglas MacArthur venting his views on the validity of the International Military Tribunal for the Fast East—i.e. the Tokyo war crimes trials—letters that contained sharp criticism of America's occupation policy. My father's diary, together with these other materials, was subsequently published in four volumes under the title *Sugamo nikki*, revised and edited by Professor Emeritus Takashi Ito of the University of Tokyo. The work has also appeared in an abridged English version, titled *Sugamo Diary*, published in the United Kingdom by Hurst Publishers.

Through these materials one also gets a clear picture of my father's sentiments as he passed the days in Sugamo Prison. He was driven, almost to distraction, by the dual desires to dedicate his life to praying for the repose of the souls of all those, Japanese and non-Japanese alike, whose lives had been sacrificed in World War II, and to establish perpetual peace on Earth. He put these sentiments into practice immediately after his release from Sugamo.

From a zealous patriot second to none in prewar days, after the war my father, adopting an unquenchable humanitarian spirit, became a relentless advocate of "world peace", not just for the sake of Japan but for the good of America and people the world over. Those who knew my father before the war looked upon the transformed Ryoichi Sasakawa as a hypocrite, or at the very least they took a cool view of his "conversion" from being an ultra-nationalist. My father had by no means undergone a conversion, however, and much less was he a hypocrite.

Critical biographies and scholarly monographs based on my father's words and actions before, during and after World War II have already well demonstrated that in both prewar and postwar days my father consistently acted, without contradiction, in accordance with his guiding principle of global humanitarianism. In fact, it is from that guiding principle that he created his now familiar motto: "The World Is One Family; Human Beings Are All Brothers and Sisters."These words appear in his diary as early as 1939. Other messages my father always directed to the world include "Japan exists thanks to the world, and we each exist thanks to Japan" and "Humankind is a family riding on Spaceship Earth".

As I will describe later, in 1962 my father established the Japan Shipbuilding Industry Foundation to support Japan's postwar recovery, and in the TV commercials made for this organization, in which he personally appeared, he always quoted this favoured slogan of his. As a result, virtually no Japanese alive at the time is unfamiliar with this motto—that's how famous it became.

The Japanese media, however, failed to understand my father's true intentions, instead baselessly and persistently portraying him as a villain. But no matter how much the media might speak evil of him, my father never attempted to defend himself against their aspersions. When asked why, he replied that newspaper and magazine journalists too had to make a living, and he felt it would be wrong if they were to lose their jobs because of him.

My father often said that any person who embraced a desire to be highly regarded during his lifetime was incapable of doing anything worthy of such an opinion. My father lived his life in the traditional mould of a true Japanese male: holding firm to his convictions, always acting in accordance with his conscience, never attempting to refute criticism no matter what the circumstances might demand. For these traits of his, I always held my father in the highest esteem.

In keeping with his words, my father dedicated the second half of his life to performing humanitarian deeds on the global stage—especially the fight against leprosy. His unwavering passion and capacity to take action moved, and were greeted with appreciation by, local people wherever he went, others involved in his causes, statesmen and social activists alike. It is for these reasons that, within the global community, the work accomplished by Ryoichi Sasakawa is held in high regard.

Back in Japan, though, my father remained a target of the media's scathing criticism, and even the philanthropic work he performed using his personal assets was looked upon with a suspicious eye.

Why was my father invariably subjected to such treatment? I have always felt that Ryoichi Sasakawa must rank among the individuals of the postwar era most discriminated against—a conclusion I inevitably reach whenever I ponder my father's life, the path he walked. What's more, the "discrimination" against him continues today, more than twenty years after his death. Even now the slander against my father, replete with misunderstanding and prejudice, goes on, negating any hope of his ever receiving a truly fair and just appraisal.

In the many years since I decided to carry on my father's lifelong commitment to eliminating leprosy, I have personally witnessed the unspeakably harsh prejudice and discrimination long suffered by people affected by leprosy, and the fight they have waged against these injustices. And in the process of seeing at first hand how they have fought their battle, I have come to believe that I must take on another personal mission: to address the prejudice and discrimination inflicted on my father.

I also believe I have a lifelong commitment to continuing with research and publishing activities to convey, correctly, what my father did during his lifetime for the sake of both Japan and the world at large. Leprosy is a disease long seen as punishment for evil done in a previous life. And while this may differ in form from the baseless discrimination that was suffered by my father, Ryoichi Sasakawa, I cannot set aside the feeling deep within me that underlying both of these "scourges" lurks an issue relating to our human nature: the propensity to discriminate against one's fellow human beings.

Motorboat racing and postwar recovery

The Nippon Foundation traces its origins to the establishment of the Japan Shipbuilding Industry Foundation, an organization created in 1962 and tasked with collecting a portion of the proceeds from domestic motorboat racing and using it for the benefit not just of Japan but of the entire world. In 2011, in line with revisions made to the nation's legal framework, the Japan Shipbuilding Industry Foundation received authorization as a public-interest incorporated foundation, whereupon its name was changed to the Nippon Foundation. The name change notwithstanding, the fundamental aim of the organization remains to conduct humanitarian activities around the world applying proceeds from Japan's boat racing industry.

It was my father who introduced motorboat racing into Japan. How and why did he come to focus on this sport?

My father is on record as having stated that it all came about as the direct result of his seeing, by chance, photographs of motorboats in a copy of *Life* magazine during his confinement at Sugamo Prison. He surreptitiously took the photos from this American publication with him when he was released from prison.

This in itself doesn't adequately answer the question as to why he focused on motorboat racing. It's not even known, for example, where he got the notion of using the proceeds from boat racing to perform a host of humanitarian activities. I myself am completely in the dark on this point, and unfortunately I never asked my father about the details that led to his decision. At this point, all one can do is to speculate on the basis of what he wrote on the matter and so on, and my conjecture is as follows.

After the war drew to its close, my father felt it was now his mission in life to do something for those whose lives had been sacrificed in the war, as well as to promote world peace and the salvation of humankind. What he ultimately aspired to was more than simply becoming a private philanthropist. Japan in those days was universally disparaged as a nation guilty of war crimes, and my father believed that the best way of restoring the country's dignity would be to make positive contributions to the world through humanitarian activities. This way of thinking was only natural in the light of my father's lifelong motto that "Japan exists thanks to the world, and we each exist thanks to Japan".

Japan at the time hardly had the wherewithal to consider undertaking humanitarian deeds on the world's behalf, however. The country lay in ruins in the wake of the war and its people were constantly scrambling to find their next meal. The matter needing to be addressed first was thus the recovery of Japanese industry.

When my father was young he had an avid interest in aeroplanes and the aviation industry. Early on he aspired to become a pilot, and even after he became independently wealthy, in a private capacity he built an airport and donated it to Japan together with a dozen or more trainer aircraft. It is only conjecture, but I imagine that my father may have first set his sights not on boat racing but on the aviation industry. This was near to impossible to achieve at the time, given that Japan was still under occupation and was forbidden to develop an aircraft industry. Developing a shipping industry, on the other hand, was feasible because there was no interdiction against it. Above all, Japan, being an archipelago, is surrounded by ocean waters, and in prewar days it had a thriving shipbuilding industry of a global nature, so the country had advantages in terms of both human resources and experience. So long as national recovery went forward smoothly, it should be more than feasible for the country to recover on the basis of its strengths in shipbuilding and shipping—and to my father, boat racing probably seemed one potential means to that end.

Once industrial recovery has been achieved, the next question that arises is how to make contributions to "promote world peace and the salvation of humankind". This, I am sure, is how my father thought at the time: "Maybe it would be possible, for example, for Japan's shipbuilding and shipping industries to pool funds for that purpose; or, even better, maybe it would be possible to create a new mechanism of the sort that would collect money to be directly applied to undertaking philanthropic activities."

I imagine these are the thoughts that continuously went through my father's mind as he passed his days at Sugamo Prison. And this is why, when he saw those photos in *Life* magazine, he must have had a revelation of sorts. For only two months after he was released from incarceration, my father began working energetically toward enacting what eventually became known as the Motorboat Racing Act. In this way, an inspiration engendered by a chance glance at some photos in a foreign magazine developed into a very specific plan by the time my father regained his personal freedom.

The Motorboat Racing Act and the Japan Shipbuilding Industry Foundation

Ever since 11 March 2011, the fateful day when Japan suffered enormous devastation as a result of the Great East Japan Earthquake and ensuing tsunami, I have often wondered what went through my father's mind in those days—"those days" referring to the latter half of the 1940s, a period when Japan, having lost the war, laboured under the cataclysmic destruction of many of its cities, Tokyo included, and much of its population was hungry or starving.

For several months after the earthquake disaster, TV coverage showed over and over the complete devastation that had been wrought by the tsunami to the area along the Pacific coast in the Tohoku region. And whenever I watched these painful scenes unfold on the screen, I was reminded of the scenes of Tokyo I had witnessed as a child, the city reduced to ashes from relentless air-bombing, and of the days when, having lost everything in those air raids, my mother and I lived in uncertainty of what tomorrow might bring. I imagine that my father too, in the aftermath of the war, had felt the same—or, more likely, an even greater—overpowering sense of impatience to "do" something to make the situation better.

What would be needed to put Japan back on its feet and lift the Japanese people out of their dire circumstances? Above all, it would take money. National recovery would require a vast amount of money. And as a viable source of the needed funds, my father hit upon the idea of boat racing, a sport that had not yet arrived in Japan.

Once he had his intention set, he wasted no time in moving forward. In February 1949, less than two months after he was released from Sugamo

Prison, my father went to the Ministry of Transport with a proposal that he himself had drafted for a law that would eventually be known as the Motorboat Racing Act. Under Japan's penal code, gambling of any kind was forbidden in those days, so before boat racing could be turned into a business it was necessary first to create a new legal framework. Two forms of "public sports"—competitive sports for which parimutuel betting was legal—did already exist, operating under government auspices. Horseracing had been reintroduced in 1946, and bicycle races had been authorized since 1948 under the Bicycle Racing Act. Records reveal that international boat racing competitions between Japan and the United States were held in Tokyo (Edogawa) and Kanagawa Prefecture (Zushi) in 1950, drawing large crowds of enthusiastic viewers. In this way, my father's plan was well suited to the times, years when the Japanese people were craving recreation and amusement.

My father energetically took his proposal to political leaders and wherever else appropriate, and as a result of these ardent efforts, in 1951 a bill was put forward by Diet members for the body's consideration during its regular session. On that occasion, three reasons were cited for proposing the bill: motorboat racing's potential contribution to the development of Japan's shipping industry, to serve as an underlying basis for national economic development; racing's useful role in spreading the conviction that without a shipping industry Japan would be unable to develop, coupled with the stimulation of tourism; and racing's contribution to local government coffers.

The bill was passed in the House of Representatives, but in the House of Councillors it met opposition from the Japan Socialist Party and was rejected. The defeat was due to the increasingly serious social problem at the time of family breakdowns caused by excessive gambling on bicycle races. Numerous cases were becoming known of families losing all their assets to gambling, and the prevailing opinion in the upper chamber questioned the wisdom of approving any new forms of public betting on competitive sports.

My father refused to lose hope, however, and he tirelessly went to meet with every representative he could, attempting to win them over and have them back the passage of the bill. As a result of these indefatigable efforts, the bill was taken up for consideration again by the Lower House at its regular session on the very last day of the current session of the Diet. It passed once again, and in line with Japanese parliamentary protocol, the vote of confirmation resulted in the bill's formal enactment and promulgation on 18 June. Just how exceptional this turn of events was can be understood from the fact that it marked the first time in the history of constitutional government in Japan that a bill initially rejected by the House of

Councillors and sent back to the House of Representatives was there again approved, and thus ultimately passed by the nation's lawmakers. In this way motorboat racing was officially approved as a new form of publicly managed sports gambling.

The question remained, however, whether or not motorboat racing had real potential to thrive as an industry. There were many sceptics—and their doubts were well within reason, for at the time motorboat racing in fact did not exist as a professional sport anywhere on the planet. As it turned out, the sceptics' concerns were not unfounded. When motorboat racing was launched, initial sales and numbers of visitors to the race venues were well short of expectations, and for the first several years operations languished in the red. To assuage the misgivings of local governments which were becoming hesitant to continue the races, my father visited them and even promised that if the races failed to show profits, he would provide his own personal funds to compensate for any losses—and in this way he convinced them to continue the races. My father had amassed a considerable amount of money through the stock market and commodities trading, and he was determined to see boat racing get on track as a viable industry even if it meant injecting all his private wealth.

It wasn't long before his wishes began to be fulfilled. As the Japanese economy started recovering by leaps and bounds, sales revenue from boat racing rose steadily. From roughly 2.4 billion yen in 1952, in the span of just ten years gross sales reached some 48 billion yen in 1962—an increase by a factor of about twenty. Nevertheless a great deal of time was still necessary before the motorboat industry would get on track in the true sense and win social approval.

In 1953, at the request of GHQ a delegation led by Carl Shoup, an expert on tax law, undertook a study of Japan's tax system and wrote up a report of its findings. Until that time 3% of revenues from motorboat racing had been paid into the nation's coffers, but starting in 1954 the Government declared its intention to put an end to this practice. Ostensibly the change was due to advice given by Shoup, but it is said that the Government was in fact worried over criticism of directly taking money generated by gambling.

What emerged from these events was legislation, to be effective for a specified duration, setting temporary exceptions to the Bicycle Racing Act and other such laws. Under this legislation part of the revenues from the various forms of publicly managed gambling were to be paid not to the Government but to specified recipient groups; the recipients in turn were required to use the funds to extend loans or provide subsidies for the purpose of promoting the nation's machine industry. The same legislation also limited the number of races that were to be allowed.

The exceptional legislation enacted at that time was also epoch-making in the sense that it stated clearly, for the very first time, that part of the revenues generated by boat racing could be applied to operations of a promotional nature. The various promotional works undertaken today by the Nippon Foundation can trace their origins to this time.

The conflict between public opinion and promotion of industry, on the one hand, and the argument in favour of terminating all publicly managed sports gambling, on the other, continued until finally, in 1962, Japan's racing laws were revised and boat racing was approved as a permanent undertaking. Coinciding with this legal revision, a new body was created to handle the proceeds from racing operations earmarked for allocation for various purposes: the Japan Shipbuilding Industry Foundation, precursor of today's Nippon Foundation.

My father's humanitarian activities and encounter with leprosy

The motorboat racing proceeds collected by the Japan Shipbuilding Industry Foundation (JSIF) were initially used to fund the recovery and development of Japan's shipbuilding and shipping industries devastated as a result of the war. By their nature, the shipbuilding and shipping industries require vast amounts of capital investment, technological development and training of human resources, and the achievements registered by the JSIF in this period are well known by people in those industries.

As its operations stabilized and proceeds increased, the scope of the JSIF's activities expanded into a number of new areas: operations to support health and sanitation needs, operations relating to fire-fighting and disaster prevention, and operations to eradicate hunger and sickness on a global scale. Whether my father had envisioned that the JSIF's activities would diversify to such an extent cannot be known, but to me the notion of actively working to obliterate global hunger and sickness is perfectly in keeping with my father's pledge to devote himself to the causes of "world peace" and "the salvation of humankind".

The humanitarian activities undertaken by my father spanned a broad spectrum. The list runs long: refugee relief around the world, agricultural support to alleviate food shortages in Africa (Sasakawa Global 2000), bringing medical interns from China to university hospitals in Japan (a hundred each year) in order to raise the level of medical care in that country, support of cancer research and measures to deal with HIV and AIDS, welfare for the elderly and disabled, and so on.

In all situations my father never wasted time coming to a decision. "Act first, then think," he always taught me. Whenever he saw someone in dire straits of whatever sort, he felt an inner compulsion to do something on their behalf. Later in life I came to view this quality of his as "the feeling of distress" inherent in Eastern philosophy. (A discussion of this compassionate motivating force is a central theme of *Bushido: The Soul of Japan*, a classic work by Inazo Nitobe, first published in 1900.)

My father always extended support with speed and without hesitancy, large sums of money being provided without his setting any preconditions whatsoever. At the same time, he always exercised caution and good planning in his philanthropic endeavours, never misjudging the essence of the issue at hand. Applying these astute skills, he proceeded to carry out a succession of significant projects targeting social reform: in Africa, for example, bringing aid to refugees and raising food production efficiency in order to alleviate hunger. Many of the projects undertaken by my father have subsequently been carried on, by the Nippon Foundation. My father possessed great powers of foresight.

The project to which my father devoted himself more than all others was the cure of patients with leprosy, marked by activities toward obliterating the disease itself. This battle against leprosy truly occupied the second half of his life.

As I will describe in detail below, it was in this connection that he set up a new organization called the Sasakawa Memorial Health Foundation (SMHF). From the outset, the foundation developed a close relationship with the World Health Organization, and carried out activities in support of leprosy-endemic nations around the world.

Whenever my father went overseas to visit developing countries for other reasons, he always made a point whenever possible to visit leprosariums. Here, he would talk to patients individually, hold their hands, and offer them encouragement. On occasions he would also eat with them. What he tried to show at first hand is that if we have correct knowledge about leprosy, then we know that we can have direct contact with leprosy patients, demonstrating that leprosy is not a disease we need be afraid of.

Why was my father so passionate about leprosy? What made him decide to dedicate his life to the eradication of leprosy? Leprosy isn't the only disease in this world that poses a threat to humankind, so why did he choose to focus on leprosy? These are questions that may be gnawing away in many people's minds. And frankly, I too long harboured these questions, prompting me to ask my father for answers. His response was quite simple. What inspired him went something like this.

When my father was young, he fell in love with a beautiful girl who lived nearby. She appears to have been my father's first love in life. One day the girl suddenly vanished—and rumour had it that she had contracted leprosy.

As I described earlier, in Japan in those days leprosy was not only feared as an incurable hereditary disease, but in a religious context it was considered a defilement, with Buddhism viewing leprosy as an inevitable punishment for evil deeds in an earlier life. As such, if any member of a family came down with leprosy, the family—and the entire extended family, too—became a target of discrimination. Marriage to such a person was, as one might expect, forbidden.

The girl who was the object of my father's affections knew this, and in her overwhelming sorrow she left home and went missing.

Her disappearance, and the conditions that drove her to it, dealt my father, still a young man, a heavy blow. And at the same time he appears to have grown angry as well. The person who contracts leprosy isn't at fault, so why must he or she be a target of such discrimination and ostracism? It was this experience in his youth that created my father's determination to some day defeat this disease, this scourge known as leprosy.

Some people may wonder if this one experience in his youth was the entire motivation behind my father's creation of what became such a large organization. To such doubts I would answer that when a human being sets his or her mind to dedicating life to a particular cause, often such a decision is based on a personal experience or motivation of this kind. And this was especially so in the case of my father, a man of strong resolution and action.

In this anecdote from his past I sense the kind of "righteous indignation" so characteristic of Ryoichi Sasakawa. For my father, the fight against leprosy was a fight against discrimination—and a fight based on his righteous indignation against discrimination.

Here I would like to introduce the relationship between my father and Yasunari Kawabata (1899–1972), the Japanese writer who won the Nobel Prize for Literature in 1968, and the unlikely ties between these two men and leprosy.

When my father and Kawabata were in primary school, their fathers were rivals in the game of Go, so as children they became friends and often visited each other's homes. After graduation, my father was advised by his school principal not to pursue higher education, and he was sent away to a Buddhist temple. Kawabata, on the other hand, proceeded to secondary school and then on to Tokyo Imperial University, where he entered the Faculty of Literature. In this way, these two childhood playmates ultimately travelled very different life paths: one a patriotic youth in Osaka, a commercial city in western Japan, the other a young lad enamoured of literature living in the bustling capital of Tokyo in eastern Japan.

In prewar years Kawabata made the acquaintance of a young man who was living in isolation at Tama Zenshoen, a leprosarium located on the outskirts of Tokyo. Kawabata provided moral support to this young man, an aspiring writer named Tamio Hojo. He also offered guidance of a professional nature and supported the publication of Hojo's first work, a novella titled *Inochi no shoya* (The First Night of Life). Even today this work is acclaimed as a masterpiece not only of "leprosy literature" but as a penetrating examination of human existence itself.

In those years it was still believed, and greatly feared, that one could contract leprosy merely by touching the belongings of a leprosy patient. This makes it all the more exceptional for the times that Kawabata should demonstrate such kindness to Hojo. Kawabata and my father sought different paths in life, but Kawabata, like my father, was a man of strong convictions who refused to be tainted by the prejudices and discriminatory views held by the world at large. Kawabata too was a man born with "the feeling of distress" which traditionally helped define a noble and honourable "true" Japanese.

Child playmates though they were, Yasunari Kawabata and Ryoichi Sasakawa had entirely different philosophies and ways of life, and yet, through their respective connections with leprosy perhaps, they felt a strong kindred spirit and renewed their old friendship. In the same way, through my father I cannot but feel mysterious connections with Yasunari Kawabata and with Tamio Hojo, a writer who ultimately went to a very early death.

Birth of the Sasakawa Memorial Health Foundation

An undertaking on a global scale launched by two septuagenarians

The pledge made by my father in his young years—to defeat leprosy once and for all—shifted into action in the 1960s, in two ways. First, my father determined to construct facilities for leprosy patients overseas—ultimately, fourteen facilities in eight countries. He also resolved to construct and improve leprosariums within Japan.

As I described in Chapter 1, however, Japan's Leprosy Prevention Law was revised in 1953 and remained on the books at that time, meaning that leprosy patients were still being forcibly isolated in sanatoriums and had no choice but to live out their lives there—a clear violation of their human rights. Abroad, meanwhile, several million leprosy patients were suffering the ravages of their disease and were also exposed to social and religious prejudice and discrimination.

It was against this backdrop that my father, anguishing over whether there wasn't something he could possibly do to alleviate these deplorable circumstances, made the acquaintance of Morizo Ishidate, Professor Emeritus of the University of Tokyo. As I related in Chapter 1, Professor Ishidate was the first person in Japan to successfully synthesize the leprosy drug promin. Today he is often referred to as the "father of chemotherapy in Japan".

My father met Professor Ishidate in May 1973 at a luncheon held at a restaurant then located within the JSIF building. The lunch meeting had been organized to decide the future directions of the Life Planning Centre, an incorporated foundation that had just been inaugurated to address matters pertaining to preventive medicine. There were five participants present: Dr. Shigeaki Hinohara, who was my father's regular doctor; Kenzo Kiikuni, who later became the SMHF chair; Professor Ishidate; my father; and me.

The Life Planning Centre Foundation remains active today, and Dr. Hinohara served as chairperson until his death in 2017, at the age of 105. Today the importance of preventive medicine is common knowledge, but when the foundation was created in 1973 preventive medicine was an innovative notion in Japan.

Professor Ishidate took part in the meeting for this new foundation in view of his role as a core member, together with Dr. Hinohara, of the Japan Overseas Christian Medical Cooperative Service (JOCS). He issued a proposal to those assembled, asking for their endorsement of the foundation's activities focused on leprosy overseas, especially its medical care being offered in Southeast Asia.

"In the modern era, measures to address leprosy in Japan got under way with the assistance of missionaries and philanthropists from abroad," Professor Ishidate told those present. "Today, Japan has joined the ranks of the advanced industrial nations, but when it comes to helping the developing countries, where measures to fight leprosy are lagging and people are still suffering, don't you find it strange that Japan is doing nothing? Sasakawa-san, it is our obligation, and a matter of honour, for Japan to aid leprosy patients overseas, don't you agree?" Everyone in attendance was moved by Professor Ishidate's proposal and offered their immediate endorsement.

To undertake medical activities overseas would require an enormous budget, though, and there was concern that the newly inaugurated Life Planning Centre would be incapable of performing the necessary activities adequately. In response to these apprehensions, my father immediately suggested that another new foundation be created specifically for that purpose. Thus the wheels were suddenly and swiftly set in motion to form what became the Sasakawa Memorial Health Foundation, tasked with performing medical activities targeting leprosy overseas.

At the time, Professor Ishidate was seventy-two years of age and my father was seventy-four. These two septuagenarians thus came to form the core of what they proclaimed would become a grand undertaking on a global scale. In retrospect, the meeting of these two men was an event of tremendous significance.

Until that time my father's leprosy-related activities had consisted primarily of improving the living environments at facilities that dealt with leprosy patients and people affected by leprosy. But now, having secured a most worthy partner in the "father of chemotherapy in Japan", I believe my father came to realize a new possibility: that perhaps leprosy itself might be eradicable from the world. Professor Ishidate, upon making my father's acquaintance, simultaneously acquired the opportunity to realize his long-cherished dream: to carry out his work to eliminate leprosy on a global scale—a prospect that surely made his enthusiasm and determination burn even brighter.

I believe my father and Professor Ishidate—men both born in the Meiji era, the period, beginning in 1868, when Japan emerged from three centuries of feudalism—had many points in common. First, they didn't talk about what had transpired in the past; rather, they both focused only on the future, and always with a positive attitude. Second, both men were burning with a sense of mission and an extremely strong determination to bring their mission to fruition.

Both my father and Professor Ishidate, even in their seventies, remained full of vigour, men who embraced their dreams with great passion. Humans can be in their prime at any age. This is why today, in addition to my father, I look up to Professor Ishidate and Dr. Hinohara as my mentors in the fine art of living.

Working closely with national governments: a new approach

The Sasakawa Memorial Health Foundation was formally approved on May 4, 1974. At the time of its official founding, the SMHF's Board of Directors consisted of ten members, with Ryoichi Sasakawa in the position of chairman and Professor Ishidate serving as board chairman. Board members included Dr. Hinohara; Shigetaka Takashima, head of the Nagashima Aiseien national sanatorium in Okayama Prefecture; Kazuchika Shiga, head of the Kikuchi Keifuen national sanatorium in Kumamoto Prefecture; Kazuo Saikawa, head of the Okinawa Airakuen national sanatorium; and Kenzo Kiikuni, who at the time was affiliated to the former National Institute of Health Services Management. Later, a growing list of highly motivated experts joined, including Suminori Tsurusaki, chief secretary of the Oku-Komyoen national sanatorium in Okayama Prefecture, who became the SMHF's first general secretary. In this way, the SMHF attracted a steadily expanding array of supporters, leading to the development of an international network of human resources.

Another individual who, by a quirk of fate, came to participate in the SMHF's leprosy activities was Dr. Yo Yuasa, former president of the International Leprosy Association (ILA). Dr. Yuasa continued to serve as an advisor to the SMHF until his retirement in 2012.

Dr. Yuasa's father was Hachiro Yuasa, first president of the International Christian University (ICU) in Tokyo and a renowned collector of Japanese folk crafts. Yo Yuasa contracted tuberculosis when he was young and spent a lengthy amount of time in hospital, an experience that inspired him to become a doctor who could empathize with his patients. To carry out his aspiration he went to the United States to study, but a relapse of tuberculosis made him abandon his plans to become a physician. Later, he resolved instead to become a psychologist and was planning to return to the United States when a friend, a patient at Nagashima Aiseien, pleaded with him to teach English to the sanatorium's inmates. Yuasa agreed, and setting aside his intention to study abroad he became an English teacher at this island sanatorium in the Inland Sea.

In 1958 the International Congress of Leprology convened in Tokyo, and through the Japanese Leprosy Foundation (Tofu Kyokai) Yuasa was engaged to help the organizers prepare for the conference and afterwards produce the transactions of the proceedings. Through these experiences and the people he met, he learned a great deal about leprosy and decided to make it his career. First, however, he was advised to get a medical degree and went to study medicine at the University of Edinburgh in Scotland. After graduating, he worked a further five years in the UK as a doctor, and did a year's training in tropical medicine, before being hired by the Leprosy Mission to go and work in Nepal in 1973.

Years later, Dr. Yuasa told me that at the time of his assignment he was prepared to spend the rest of his life in Nepal doing leprosy-related fieldwork. Nepal in those days was one of the countries with a heavy burden of leprosy.

In 1974 Dr. Yuasa, representing Nepal, attended an international seminar on leprosy control cooperation in Asia organized by the SMHF in Oiso, Kanagawa Prefecture. Dr. Yuasa later told me that although he undertook his work in Nepal in those days with lofty ambition, locally his work had met with considerable resistance and he felt as if he had run up against a brick wall. It was while in Oiso that he saw the innovative approach SMHF was taking to leprosy work, and, backed by the recommendation of his British mentor, he decided to return to Japan and participate in SMHF's activities.

Why was Dr. Yuasa so attracted to SMHF—to the extent that he chose to abandon his plan to devote his entire life to fieldwork in Nepal? He said he appreciated the foundation's modus operandi, which emphasized building relationships with the health authorities of leprosy-endemic countries and helping them strengthen their leprosy control strategies—an approach that his role in Nepal did not permit him to pursue.

SMHF's approach stemmed from a philosophy espoused by Professor Ishidate, who always stressed that, while SMHF's work should have a humanitarian aspect, it should be based on scientific and public health principles. That being the case, it saw support for national governments as the only way to deal with leprosy in public health terms, in contrast to the approach that other NGOs tended to adopt at that time in pursuing their own projects.

In the beginning, reaction to this policy adopted by the foundation was not always positive. "Why do you want to work with national governments everywhere?" we were asked. "Don't you know that governments in developing countries are unstable and can't be trusted? Wouldn't you get better results by dealing directly with the patients?" But SMHF's members—including Professor Ishidate, Dr. Yuasa, who had real experience in the medical care of leprosy overseas, and Dr. Saikawa, who had conducted outpatient treatment of leprosy within Japan—were firmly convinced, based on their experience, that dealing with patients alone would not suffice.

Happily, in recent years, as the policies and achievements of SMHF have come to be acknowledged, the importance and effectiveness of liaising with stakeholders from all quarters, and especially with national governments, have become widely recognized.

Relationship with WHO built on trust

What has been important in making SMHF's work more effective has been the close working relationship it developed with the World Health Organization (WHO). Here, I would like to describe how the SMHF came to form its strong ties with the WHO.

At six o'clock one morning in 1975, the year after the SMHF was founded, my father made an impromptu phone call to Kenzo Kiikuni, a member of the Board of Directors. He took Professor Kiikuni utterly by surprise by telling him that he wanted to donate $1 million to countries in Africa experiencing difficulties relating to leprosy, and he enquired how he might go about doing so.

"Even if you were to give money directly to the countries of Africa," Professor Kiikuni responded, "I doubt it would be used effectively for the benefit of people with leprosy. What I would suggest instead is to provide the funds to the WHO, an international organization involved in health care issues around the world, and have them work up a plan." My father thought this was a good idea.

"So where is this WHO located?" my father asked.

"In Geneva, Switzerland."

"Then please go immediately, tomorrow, to Geneva and discuss this matter with the WHO."

Today, in retrospect, this anecdote brings a smile to the professor's face, but he says he was flabbergasted by how my father operated—the way he made such instant and utterly bold decisions. On the surface, the way he did things may seem quite rash; but it goes without saying that my father was fully aware of Professor Kiikuni's capabilities as an expert and had complete faith in entrusting his daring mission to him.

One month later, Professor Kiikuni, accompanied by Professor Ishidate and Dr. Saikawa, went to Geneva and met with the then Director-General of the WHO, Dr. Halfdan Mahler. In those days leprosy was already becoming a "forgotten disease" at the WHO, but upon hearing of my father's offer Dr. Mahler immediately responded that he would eagerly accept it as a way of once again addressing leprosy as an issue of great importance.

The contingent from the SMHF returned to Tokyo in high spirits. It wasn't long thereafter that Professor Kiikuni received another early morning phone call—this time from Dr. Mahler at four o'clock, the unlucky result of a mistake in judging the time difference. "Today the WHO is at a vital juncture in its fight to eliminate smallpox," the Director-General began, "and we were wondering if we might be allowed to use even part of the money Mr. Sasakawa is donating for the cause of smallpox." At the time, the final battles toward eradication of smallpox were being fought in Somalia and Ethiopia, but because both countries were embroiled in civil war, the WHO assumed that considerable costs would be involved in transporting the smallpox vaccine to where it was needed most.

Professor Kiikuni immediately went to discuss the matter with my father. My father listened to the message in silence, and then asked one question: "Is this Dr. Mahler a man who can be trusted?"

"I've only met the man once," the professor replied, but he then went on to relate to my father what Dr. Mahler had told him in Geneva of his personal background: that he was the son of a Danish pastor, that for many years he had served as a medical specialist in tuberculosis in Central America and India, doing volunteer work without regard for the dangers lurking around him, and so on. "I think he's a man who can be trusted," he concluded.

"OK, now I understand," my father responded. "Please tell Dr. Mahler that the money I've donated was given to him. Tell him that he may use it freely in whatever way he feels it would be put to best use."

When Professor Kiikuni phoned Dr. Mahler with my father's message, he was deeply moved. "We've never before had anyone donate a sum as great as a million dollars and not specify exactly how it was to be used," he confessed. "I give you my word, one day I will come to Japan myself to convey my appreciation to Mr. Sasakawa." As promised, two years later Dr. Mahler came to meet my father and present him with the WHO's certificate of appreciation. After that first meeting, he proceeded to visit Japan on frequent occasions, always taking time to meet with my father and deepen their relationship.

It was five years after my father made his donation that the WHO issued a global declaration, in 1980, of having eradicated smallpox. My father's financial aid had played a significant role during the final stages of eradicating the disease, with the result that even now the WHO speaks of the debt it owes to my father for his help in ridding the world of smallpox. A bust of my father has been installed at the WHO's Geneva headquarters, and bus guides tell Japanese tourists of the deeds he accomplished.

In reminiscing about those days, Professor Kiikuni confessed to me that before he actually met my father, all he knew about him was what people gossiped—that he was a right-wing boss and so on. "But after I began working with him on our activities," he related, "on many occasions I came to see what a truly capable and magnanimous man he was. He could see through a person in an instant, or win a person over in an instant too. And he could also stir people to action, no doubt because of all the hellishness he himself had gone through. Everyone who worked with him, creating and supporting the foundation, including Professor Ishidate and Dr. Saikawa, trusted your father from the depths of their hearts."

Without question, my father was a genius at rousing people to action. He was also a genius capable of forming solid ties of mutual trust with others, from the depths of their hearts, with others. Perhaps calling one's own father a genius sounds too boastful. If so, then let me put it this way. More than anyone on this planet my father had a pure and powerful desire to eradicate leprosy from the world, without any self-interest, desire for personal gain or unsavoury intention whatsoever. It was to his pure nature, I think, that people were attracted most.

Personal relationships of trust, an essential element
of international activities

Thanks to our involvement in leprosy issues since 1974, more than forty years ago, today virtually anyone who attends a WHO assembly is familiar with the Nippon Foundation and the Sasakawa Memorial Health Foundation. (The only people perhaps unfamiliar with our organizations are individuals who have been newly appointed to their positions.)

I myself have been involved with leprosy issues for more than forty years. As a result, whenever I attend a WHO assembly or an international forum relating to leprosy, I meet with government ministers, officials, and WHO representatives of countries from all around the world. Many such individuals are appointed to their positions for specified terms, and in a majority of instances such terms are quite short, only a few years at best. Consequently, at WHO assemblies in recent years I have made it a practice on each occasion to hire a room and use it as a venue for exchanging views on leprosy with the national health ministers in attendance. I do so out of the need to have a firm understanding of the global picture, the situation in each country, and knowledge of the people in charge in the different countries. This is so that the two foundations' work in leprosy remains in accordance with each country's specific circumstances; also, that I keep myself informed as WHO Goodwill Ambassador for Leprosy Elimination. In this sense, too, I am very proud that we have maintained a consistent complement of people in charge on our behalf, enabling us to play a significant role in working through the WHO to eliminate leprosy.

In addition—and this holds true for all international activities of every kind—another indispensable factor for ensuring smooth forward progress is ties between people: relationships of trust.

The concept of international relations conjures up in many people's minds relationships between countries or between organizations. But relying solely on relationships of these kinds can, in not a few instances, merely lead to each side stating its own position without proceeding further to a fundamental debate on the issues at stake and their resolution. To carry out this more important role requires individual relationships of trust between people.

In the course of my own international activities, I have witnessed again and again how individual relationships of trust wield a surprisingly large impact. A good example is the relationship between the Nippon Foundation and former U.S. President Jimmy Carter.

In the United States, it is customary for Presidents, once they have left office, to use public funds to construct museums, libraries and the like dedicated to their term in office. In the case of Jimmy Carter, however, the construction of an institution in his name was initially to be funded by a leading Japanese financier; but then, at the last minute, that proposal was declined. Although no clear reason was ever offered for that turn of events, the fact that Mr. Carter was succeeded by Ronald Reagan, a Republican, combined with Mr. Reagan's close relationship with Yasuhiro Nakasone, who was then serving as Japan's Prime Minister, may have raised concerns that if the Japanese financier in question were to provide funds to the preceding President, a Democrat, it might invite unnecessary misunderstanding.

Indeed, I have heard that as soon as Mr. Carter left office and a Republican administration came into power, not a few Japanese who had been close to Mr. Carter fled the scene like a rushing tide.

My father, upon hearing what had happened, immediately contacted Mr. Carter. "The Japanese are a people who keep their promises," he told the former President. "That financier must have had some circumstantial reason for what happened, so please don't think badly of him. In his stead I will provide financial assistance." And with this my father provided part of the funds needed to construct what became the Carter Center. This marked the commencement of a friendship between my father and Mr. Carter. My father even paid respects at the grave of Mr. Carter's parents, and Mr. Carter did likewise at the Sasakawa family burial site in Osaka.

In this way, my father gave financial assistance to a former U.S. President, a Democrat, who was labelled a liberal to boot, at a time when the governing administration was Republican. This also should suffice to demonstrate that Ryoichi Sasakawa was not a person who one could say in good faith fitted the simple definition of a "right-winger".

In the years since he left the presidency, Jimmy Carter has gone on to serve as a "peacemaker" on the international stage—mediating disputes in Nicaragua and Bosnia, and meeting with Kim Il-Sung to open the way for dialogue between the U.S. and North Korea. Mr. Carter has also cooperated to no small extent in the Nippon Foundation's project Sasakawa Global

2000[1], operated by the Sasakawa Africa Association(SAA), to increase food production in Africa. I might mention in passing that I myself played a small role in realizing the meeting between Mr. Carter and Kim Il-Sung, the founding father of North Korea, having discussed the possibility of their meeting on numerous occasions.

I might add here that in carrying out the Sasakawa Global 2000 initiative, another Nobel Peace Prize laureate, Dr. Norman Borlaug (1914–2009), participated as a technical advisor and expert in the Green Revolution.

At the time the project was inaugurated in 1986, Dr. Borlaug was seventy-two years of age and had already retired from all official duties. When my father approached him with a request to cooperate, he initially declined citing his age. But my father won him over with the following argument. "I'm fifteen years your senior, eighty-seven," he told Dr. Borlaug, "and I'm asking for you to work together. Isn't there a possibility of your cooperating with us?" In the face of such a persuasive argument, Dr. Borlaug could only respond in the affirmative, and indeed he must have been moved by my father's words, for later on, on numerous occasions, I heard Dr. Borlaug himself relate this anecdote at various international congresses.

Sasakawa Global 2000 scored significant successes in Africa during the 1990s. In Ethiopia, only five years after the project was launched, the country was in a position to export food.

My father volunteers to test a leprosy vaccine

The following is an anecdote indicative of my father's purity of intentions apropos the fight against leprosy.

As an adjunct to his desire to eradicate leprosy, my father had great interest in the possibility of developing a vaccine to prevent the disease. His interest arose from the appearance of bacteria resistant to dapsone (the successor to promin), the drug that until then had demonstrated effectiveness against leprosy since it was first used in the 1940s. Dapsone-resistant bacilli meant that

[1] In the late 1970s to early 1980s, a number of African countries were struggling to cope with a worsening hunger situation—none more so than Ethiopia and the Horn of Africa countries which had suffered from the ravages of famine. It was in this context that SAA dedicated itself to capacity building for public extension systems. Over time, SAA has worked with thousands of frontline extension agents (EAs) and millions of farmers in fifteen African countries to promote the use of improved agricultural technologies, covering a wide range of staple crops from maize, wheat, rice, teff, sorghum, millet, and legumes to roots and tubers.

an increasing number of patients appeared whose symptoms could not be treated with it. As efforts were made to find an alternative drug regimen, they were also directed at developing a vaccine.

With a vaccine that prevents leprosy it would become possible to suppress the disease before it had a chance to develop. The idea was identical to that behind the vaccine against smallpox developed by Edward Jenner (1749–1823). Researchers soon found potential for creating an anti-leprosy vaccine using armadillos, which are natural hosts of *Mycobacterium leprae*, the bacillus that causes leprosy.

When the very first prototype of a vaccine against leprosy was developed under the WHO's auspices (Special Programme for Research and Training in Tropical Diseases), my father, having awaited its development with bated breath, immediately volunteered to be the first person—the first "guinea pig"—to be inoculated. He contacted Dr. Tonetaro Ito of Osaka University's Research Institute for Microbial Diseases, a member of the research team, and personally conveyed his determination. "I want to demonstrate to the world that this vaccine is safe," he told Dr. Ito, "and I want to help achieve its smooth, widespread use. Please, I beg you, test the vaccine on me."

To be vaccinated for leprosy equates to having leprosy pathogens implanted within one's body. Normally, even armed with the knowledge that such a vaccination is said to be medically safe, few, if any, would ever choose to be the first human to test it.

Osaka University and the WHO were at a loss as to how they should respond. It was decided that before proceeding it would be necessary to secure approval from the ethics committees of both the university and the WHO. Approval was duly granted, and on 8 December 1987 my father became the first human in history to be inoculated with a vaccine against leprosy. The historic event took place at the WHO's headquarters in Geneva, in the presence of Director-General Mahler. More than anyone else, before the whole world my father wanted to demonstrate, for the sake of eradicating leprosy, that the newly developed vaccine was safe and nothing to be afraid of.

Thanks to the remarkable success of multidrug therapy (MDT), which became the recommended treatment in place of dapsone monotherapy from the 1980s, the prevalence of leprosy declined dramatically and for a time the need to develop a vaccine became less of a priority. In recent years, however, the number of new cases has remained consistently above 200,000. It may well be that a vaccine is one of the tools needed to defeat the disease, and efforts are now under way again to develop one.

NO MATTER WHERE THE JOURNEY TAKES ME

"I have no desire to be acclaimed by others during my lifetime," my father used to say. But on just one occasion he was more than thrilled to win recognition from someone: in 1983, when he received a personal invitation from Pope John Paul II, expressing his wish to thank my father for his many years of dedication to the eradication of leprosy.

On 9 May 1983, just days after celebrating his eighty-fourth birthday, my father was invited to the Pope's office at the Vatican. As was his wont whenever he travelled abroad, on this occasion my father dressed in formal Japanese attire: *haori-hakama*, a loose-fitting half-length jacket and wide pleated trousers.

The Pope expressed strong interest in the subject of leprosy. "You've made great contributions to humanity through your efforts to bring world peace, and especially to eradicate smallpox," His Holiness began. "And now you are making special efforts in the fight against leprosy. I want to express my appreciation for all that you are doing to eliminate suffering and inequality from the world, and I ask you, please, to continue to make greater and greater efforts in these ways in the years ahead." And as he finished, the Pope extended his two arms to my father to welcome him in his embrace.

In instances like that, a Catholic person would apparently accept the Pope's embrace in silence. My father, though, being so deeply moved by the words of appreciation expressed by His Holiness, instinctively held out his arms in a similar manner toward the Pope, a man taller than him, resulting in the two men hugging each other. Later, over dinner at our hotel in Rome, my father described the incident to me in this way: "The Pope is younger than me, yet somehow the feeling that came over me was like being embraced by my father when I was a child. I could feel His Holiness's great benevolence and powerful love." My father seemed genuinely thrilled.

I have a photo taken that day. My father, dressed in his formal black garb being embraced by Pope John Paul II in his white ceremonial robes, looks like a mischievous schoolboy with a huge smile on his face. This was my father as I had never seen him before. He had been granted more than thirty minutes in private with His Holiness; their meeting was no mere formality slipped in between other audiences. I later heard that in fact what transpired between my father and the Pope was quite rare indeed.

The level of activity maintained by Ryoichi Sasakawa, a man of action and decisive determination, did not diminish an iota even as his years grew in number. In the sixteen years between his eightieth birthday and his death at the age of ninety-six, my father travelled overseas on no fewer than 103 occasions, averaging seven or eight trips per year. Every trip he undertook in these years was to carry out humanitarian activities, including those related to leprosy.

86

"I wasn't born for the sake of my children or grandchildren," he used to say. "I was created to help the disadvantaged in this world." To this end, he worked 365 days a year, never resting even for a day. Despite the unjust misunderstanding, prejudice and discrimination that he faced, he continued to rush hither and thither for the benefit of others, casting aside all self-interest and never seeking recompense of any sort. In his long life devoted to others, he was given one reward of irreplaceable value: his meeting with Pope John Paul II. I am profoundly grateful that he was honoured with such a wondrous gift.

The Work of the Nippon Foundation

A noble public sport, or just gambling?

Today the Nippon Foundation is one of the world's largest organizations of its kind, its assets total some 278.5 billion yen (FY2017) and its annual budget run to 45.2 billion yen (FY2017). In addition to a plethora of activities undertaken within Japan—ranging from maritime and social welfare projects to the promotion of sports and tourism—the Foundation has for many years also provided sustained support to humanitarian causes on a global scale. Even today, however, criticism is voiced in some quarters toward the conduct of such aid programmes using proceeds from motorboat racing, a publicly operated competitive sport. "No matter how noble the causes for which it's used, it's still money that was made through gambling" is the typical argument. This view exists not only within Japan but is also found among grantees overseas as well.

All money, of whatever provenance, has equal value. The issue, I believe, is how it is used. In the case of the funds employed by the Nippon Foundation to conduct its diverse activities, their origins can be traced to every 100 or 200 yen spent by fans of motorboat racing to enjoy their preferred form of recreation. This is why I firmly believe that at the Nippon Foundation we have an obligation whenever we apply our financial resources, in no matter how small an amount, to always use them responsibly.

Many people, even today, are under the mistaken impression that the Nippon Foundation is the operator of the nation's motorboat racing industry. This misconception is surely where the criticism of our being a "bookmaker" stems from. Such criticism does not comport with the facts, however. The Motorboat Racing Law of Japan states clearly that the nation's motorboat races are to be operated by local public bodies; moreover, the races themselves are run by the Japan Motor Boat Racing Association—an organization altogether separate from the Nippon Foundation.

Allocation of the proceeds accrued from the nation's boat racing industry is conducted as follows (as of 2018). First, 75% of all sales revert to the fans who bet on the races. Of the remaining 25%, approximately 2.8% is granted to the Nippon Foundation, and 1.3% paid to the Japan Motor Boat Racing Association in the form of management fees; these various allocations are all strictly regulated under law and relevant regulations. The rest becomes the revenue of the local public bodies. As this demonstrates, the motorboat racing industry has an extremely high level of transparency. In addition, the Nippon Foundation's own financial statements, business reports and the like are all made openly available for viewing on its website—a measure taken because we believe that without such openness we would be unable to gain people's correct understanding.

Personally, I think it's somewhat narrow-minded to brand gambling per se as evil.

The French philosopher Roger Caillois (1913–1978) wrote in his book *Les Jeux et les hommes* (*Man, Play and Games*) that play is at the core of all human activities. He argues that all play invariably takes one of four forms: agon (competition), alea (chance), mimicry (role playing) and ilinx (altering perception). The Dutch historian Johan Huizinga (1872–1945), writing in his *Homo Ludens* (literally, "Playing Man"), argued that humans exist to play. Taken together, these works suggest that the enjoyment of gambling is an inherent human trait—one of our most basic instincts.

Gambling does of course always have its bad sides too—namely, its attendant prodigality and speculative nature—and it is primarily for this reason that gambling has traditionally been criticized for its role in developing a quest for good fortune (and fortunes) among the masses, and in relieving them of their money. In Japanese this quest is referred to as *shakōshin*, which literally translates as "a desire to shoot down good luck". The dictionary defines *shakōshin* as the desire to gain incidental gain without effort. And when this sentiment is aroused, as critics claim, the overtone quickly becomes negative.

My father, who worked tirelessly to plant motorboat racing firmly in Japanese soil, often said that all human beings, without exception, are born with *shakōshin*. There can be no denying that it is in the human spirit to want, if chance allows, to be blessed with good fortune, and to want to get it without effort. As such, what merits admonition isn't *shakōshin*—the human desire for good fortune—but rather any act that incites it to excess.

Historically there has never been a country, at any time or anywhere, that succeeded in eradicating gambling. From this we can infer that so long as humans are born with their inherent *shakōshin*: so long as humans are human, gambling is unlikely to disappear from the face of the earth. And while there is just cause in seeking to prevent people from going to ruin by losing themselves in gambling, and in preventing antisocial elements from using gambling as a source of funds, prohibiting all gambling outright is quite unreasonable.

One answer devised to resolve this social dilemma was to permit gambling only as stipulated under the law. Another method was to employ gambling as a just way of bringing money into state coffers as a public undertaking.

In the United Kingdom, for example, a Royal Commission on gambling established in 1949 rejected the idea that gambling led to serious social and economic problems and recommended licensing and regulating it, rather than prohibiting it. This led to new gambling legislation in 1960 that legalized betting in licensed shops. Such an approach, I feel, has encouraged in the British a mature attitude to gambling.

For the sake of people who are unable to take responsibility for their own actions, should the liberty of all people be restricted; or should the aim be placed on creating a mature society in which everyone can enjoy legal gambling without losing their good sense and moderation? The various issues that surround gambling may also be an opportunity to test the discretion we can all exercise as individuals living in our times.

The work of the Nippon Foundation: from maritime support to CSR activities

In the half-century since its founding, the Nippon Foundation has consistently sought to perform works that, in response to the social demands of the times, cast light on the darker sides of society. The Foundation's earliest activities were focused on promoting Japan's shipbuilding and marine transport industries; then gradually the scope was widened from shipbuilding to maritime areas, and eventually to humanitarian activities in developing countries around the world. But as our fields of endeavour have come to span a spectrum of such remarkable breadth, it has become increasingly difficult for the average person to understand the total picture of the organization known as the Nippon Foundation. This is undeniably true. Here, therefore, I would like to present an overall introduction to the different activities undertaken by the Foundation. Broadly speaking, they divide into three major areas: maritime support, public service and volunteer work, and international cooperation.

Our maritime-related work has undergone two major shifts during the past decade or so: from a focus on ships to the seas, and from a Japan protected by the seas to a Japan that protects the seas. In particular, in line with a basic concept of passing the oceans on to future generations, we are focusing our efforts into nurturing human resources and network building, working in liaison with United Nations-affiliated organizations and the World Maritime University (WMU). Because the world's oceans and seas are all intercon-nected, encompassing individual countries' territorial waters, many maritime issues cannot be resolved by any one nation acting alone. Accordingly, culti-vating human resources and developing qualified people who are up to the tasks of formulating maritime policies and conducting marine research based on comprehensive knowledge of the oceans and seas is absolutely indispens-able. To date, the Nippon Foundation has provided maritime scholarships and fellowship grants to more than 1,060 people from 110 countries.

In addition, because it operates without individual administrative divisions or areas of specialization, the Nippon Foundation has long worked to enact a Basic Act on Ocean Policy aimed at firmly establishing maritime governance in Japan. As a result of the Foundation's approaches to the Japanese Government, the Basic Act was drawn up in 2007, followed in 2008 with the Basic Plan on Ocean Policy.

The Nippon Foundation's public service and volunteer work consists of sup-port provided to activities, locally based within Japan, in areas such as social welfare, education and culture. Examples include supporting self-reliance of the disabled, deployment of welfare vehicles, hospice programmes, healthy child rearing, environmental protection, disaster assistance, arts and culture, promo-tion of lifelong sports, and support to victims of crime. This category also includes the Foundation's support of activities focused on achieving recovery from the Great East Japan Earthquake and tsunami disaster.

A number of the Foundation's projects, as a result of having been under way for more than ten years, have come to be widely known. For over twenty years, for example, the Foundation has provided welfare vehicles for the elderly and disabled; today upwards of 40,000 vehicles are in use nationwide. For more than fifteen years up to 2013, the Foundation supported the educa-tion of palliative care nurses who assist patients with life-limiting illnesses, with some 3,700 nurses undergoing certification training.

The Nippon Foundation's activities in international cooperation consist of projects carried out in cooperation with international organizations, foreign governments, NGOs and so on, to resolve fundamental issues affecting man-kind such as poverty, starvation and sickness. Activities of this kind also encompass projects to develop human resources to perform social activities and to build related networks. Included here is our collaboration with the WHO, since 1975, to eliminate leprosy, which I have embraced as my life's work. Although little known within Japan, the Nippon Foundation is the only entity to utilize proceeds from publicly operated sports gambling in Japan for overseas grants.

Three projects stand out among the Foundation's projects involving international cooperation. First, since 1993, the Foundation has supported the construction of schools in developing countries as a way of enhancing their educational environments. Second, a scholarship programme is targeted specifically at aiding disabled persons in Asia. And third, a medical support project is under way in the developing countries that combines traditional Asian medicine with Japan's "okigusuri" system, whereby medicine boxes are provided to households, payment is made only for the amount of medicine actually used, and depleted items are regularly replenished. All of these programmes have been implemented applying the Nippon Foundation's unique perspective and methods.

Meanwhile, the Sasakawa Global 2000 programme, launched in 1986 together with Dr. Norman Borlaug and former U.S. President Jimmy Carter, provides support to agricultural projects in Africa.

In both the maritime and public service and volunteer work spheres, we have made extremely vigorous efforts to develop human resources to carry on in the next generation. In the area of international cooperation as well, in 1987 we launched the Ryoichi Sasakawa Young Leaders Fellowship Fund (Sylff) programme to develop human resources to solve various global issues. To date, fellowships have been provided to more than 15,000 graduate school students studying at 69 universities in 44 countries. The resulting pool of fellowship recipients today forms a truly dependable network of individuals able to work with the Nippon Foundation in carrying out its activities.

In addition to the foregoing, there are two other areas to which the Nippon Foundation has recently been channeling its resources: projects that cultivate a culture of donations as a way to achieve a new society, and CSR (corporate social responsibility) activities in collaboration with the corporate sector.

Today Japan has an enormous government debt exceeding 1 quadrillion yen, the result of which is an increasing number of areas where public services are inadequate. Japanese society as a whole and community life patterns are also undergoing major changes amid the nation's declining birth rate, the shift to nuclear families, a shrinking population, and depopulation of rural areas. Traditional public services—including child care support, caregiving support systems, rubbish collection and snow removal—are increasingly unable to respond to actual needs, creating a long list of issues not amenable to easy resolution.

To shed light on these issues and move closer, even modestly, toward their resolution, I believe that now, more than ever, it is essential to create a society of "people supporting people". At the same time it is also necessary to cultivate a culture of proactive donation, giving in order to support and energize the activities performed by non-profit organizations (NPOs) and volunteer networks. In addition, it will be necessary to further stimulate and add vigour to the CSR activities of the corporate sector.

In the light of the nation's social needs, in 2005 the Nippon Foundation launched a public service community website called CANPAN as a forum for information for expanding public service action networks and resolving social issues. The name CANPAN was coined from the verb "can" and the "pan" in "panacea", a remedy for all ills, literal or figurative. The website was created as a venue where NPOs can post information describing their specific activities, and also to provide a way for people who are sympathetic to an NPO's work to make donations to it online.

In 2006 the Foundation launched a second website, CANPAN CSR PLUS, where the public could browse for information relating to corporate CSR activities. CSR should be understood as a business entity's organizational strategies; but in Japan the concept became increasingly misconstrued, in a very narrow sense, equating CSR to social contributions, resulting in the loss of its original significance. CANPAN CSR PLUS was created to bring to light how companies are diligently undertaking CSR initiatives, in a quest to create opportunities to attract broad investment from abroad and energize the CSR activities of Japanese corporations.

CANPAN CSR PLUS was terminated in 2013 after having fulfilled the purposes behind its creation. Today, we are developing a consultation service for formulating a list of operations that have high social value in accordance with the phase of involvement of each corporation.

The private sector supporting the public sector: a concept both old and new

For six decades in the postwar era, the Japanese Government has told its citizens that if they work hard and pay their taxes, the Government will take full care of their social welfare needs in old age. This situation characteristic of Japanese society—the situation with which it is, in a sense, "blessed"—forms the backdrop to why the work performed by organizations like the Nippon Foundation—the private sector helping the private sector, or lending support to the public sector in helping the private sector—has for many years been inevitably limited.

Today, however, many Japanese sense deeply that those days are over. Very soon Japan will be a super-aged society. This is obvious from the nation's demographics, and as such, if no change is made to a society in which the private sector supports the private sector while also supplementing the work done by the public sector, in the not too distant future Japanese society will no longer be viable. This circumstance poses an extremely critical problem not only in the case of Japan, but also for many advanced countries facing the dual issues of a falling birthrate and an ageing population.

There are a variety of advantages to having the private sector do what only by the private sector can do. As an example, unlike national or local governments and their agencies which are tied down by regulations, the private sector is capable of free thinking and swift action. In the case of the Nippon Foundation, moreover, we have expertise and creativity cultivated through long years of activity. This is one of our greatest strengths.

Administrative institutions in particular, and other organizations of all descriptions, are said to require at least a year or a year and a half to work up a budget for a project and set the project in motion. By contrast, at the Nippon Foundation we are able to launch an aid programme in only three months or so. We accept applications for assistance at any time, and screening is performed once every three months. When necessary, if informal governmental approval must be acquired, we can provide aid immediately in cases that we have approved. This sense of speed is another feature unique to the Nippon Foundation.

Along with our ability to commence an undertaking with alacrity, a further strength is our ability, leveraging the benefits of belonging to the private sector, to provide support on a long-term and continuing basis, rather than as a one-off. The Nippon Foundation has been offering overseas aid and conducting leprosy elimination activities for roughly forty years and supporting agricultural development in Africa for close to thirty years.

The Nippon Foundation's operating policy—manifesting the vitality of the private sector to the very fullest, applying ideas of the private sector for the benefit of the private sector—traces its origins to the philosophy of my father, Ryoichi Sasakawa. When the Japan Shipbuilding Industry Foundation was founded in 1962 as the forerunner of what later became the Nippon Foundation, my father strongly opposed its treatment as a *tokushu-hōjin*: literally, a "special corporation" (a quasi-governmental corporation). As this indicates, from the outset my father was determined that the Foundation should be a private body that applied the ideas of the private sector.

My father also used to expound, whenever the occasion presented itself, on the importance of Japan's extricating itself from the abuses inherent in *kanson-minpi*—worshipping officialdom and belittling the common people—and enabling the private sector to achieve self-reliance. He believed that civil awareness in the true sense had not fully put down roots in Japan, that people continued to look up to authority, to the bureaucracy, as their foundation of dependence.

The nation's defeat in the war provided an opportune time for a major change in this public way of thinking, but the people's newfound democracy was something that had been given to them, not fought for, and this impeded the maturation of their civic awareness. After the war the bureaucrat officials who had ruled ever since the days of the Meiji period should have undergone a change to "public servants" in the literal sense, but the Japanese people ultimately were unable to give up their ingrained dependence on the bureaucracy. This is said to be the form of democracy in contemporary Japan. This aspect of Japanese society is vividly embodied, for example, in the government-dominated industrial structure of what was referred to as "Japan Inc."; in *amakudari*, the institutionalized practice of senior bureaucrats retiring to cushy jobs in industries they formerly oversaw; and in *watari*, a similar phenomenon in which retired bureaucrats flit from one job to another, each time drawing a lucrative retirement payout.

My father also always used to say that to break down this structure, it would first be necessary for the private sector to shed its dependence on the public sector. What instilled such thinking in him? I think it was the pride he took in opposing authority all his life. Motives aside, my father had correct foresight.

The conviction that, from the perspective of the private sector, light must be shed on the "dark" side of society that has been overlooked in-between laws and systems is today deeply ingrained in the organizational culture of the Nippon Foundation. And among the fruits of that position, we count how the agility and mobility unique to the private sector has, during the past fifty years, been used to maximum advantage, enabling the Nippon Foundation to apply its total resources to international cooperation such as the elimination of leprosy as well as to making social contributions within Japan.

The underlying source of the Nippon Foundation's activities and the yardstick against which we make our judgements are our set of seven Guiding Principles, principles that have been embraced ever since the Foundation was founded. Although the wording has been slightly modified from time to time in step with contemporary changes, the principles' aims have not changed from the outset. They form the very backbone of all that the Nippon Foundation aspires to do and achieve:

Discover: We identify change around the world in its earliest stages, getting quickly to work on solutions to upcoming problems that humanity will face.

Prioritize: We work constantly to understand what is needed today, and where it is required, so we can meet the needs with highest priority at all times.

Be creative: Unencumbered by precedent, we take innovative approaches to new projects, crafting fresh systems to make our society better.

Do it now: We show decisiveness and bold action, implementing our activities quickly so we can address change in real time, as it happens.

Be open: Our open stance on information disclosure allows us to listen to the voices of society, reflecting them in our actions as an always accessible organization.

Grow: We constantly keep a critical eye on ourselves, evaluating our actions and learning to improve our capacity for social innovation and the quality of our activities.

Expand networks: By extending our networks to individuals and organizations with an awareness of the problems humanity faces, we seek to create great surges of action in society.

A look at the various goals the Nippon Foundation aims to achieve, and at the various activities it pursues, shows that none are exceedingly difficult. We consider how to deal humanely with and support the social issues we see in Japan and overseas. Then we consider how to put solutions into action. And at the root of all that the Nippon Foundation does is the philosophy of its founder, Ryoichi Sasakawa: that "the world is one family; all humankind are brothers and sisters". In the final analysis, the ideals of humanitarian activities transcending differences in political views, economic situations, philosophies, religion, race and national borders all begin here.

Hub of social innovations, and beyond: the next fifty years

To create a society in which all people can live happily, it is essential for society itself to change and evolve in response to the demands of the times and of the people who make up society. And to realize such social reforms by the most preferable methods, the activities undertaken by the Nippon Foundation through the years have focused on bringing into the spotlight, and resolving, social issues that exist unseen beneath the surface.

A sampling of the most recent issues that the Nippon Foundation has successfully addressed, applying its comprehensive resources and methods that I myself devised, includes the following: enactment of the Basic Act on Ocean Policy, formation of a nationwide organization of victims of crime, creation of mechanisms to prevent criminal recidivism, encouraging more child adoptions, dealing with dormant bank accounts, and raising prices of tobacco products. The general perception of the Nippon Foundation held by the public is of an organization whose work is to provide assistance—*financial* assistance. But in fact the Nippon Foundation thinks for itself and acts on its own initiative. This is a point that separates the Nippon Foundation significantly from foundations of a general nature. That said, providing assistance to NPOs remains an important part of the Foundation's work.

My father, Ryoichi Sasakawa, often said that no matter how noble one's goal, if the result is bad then it's not worth a pittance. I adhere to this view completely. Even with the noblest of plans, if nothing is achieved from them, then the whole effort is meaningless. Any initiative once begun has to produce realistic, tangible results. I also see this as our obligation as an organization than disburses funds accrued from the public.

In October 2012, in marking its 50th anniversary the Nippon Foundation launched a new vision for the forthcoming fifty years. The vision is embodied in just three words: "social innovation hub".

In the past half-century, the parameters of social issues have changed greatly. An increasing number of issues today cannot be resolved by any nation acting alone: issues of a global nature relating to the environment, natural resources and food, for example. Meanwhile in Japan, one issue after another has come to the surface that local governments or public institutions are unable to fully address: issues such as the ageing of the population, the weakening of interpersonal relations within communities, and deterioration in childrearing environments. The power of social capital too is beginning to be called into question.

On the positive side, however, a new current—a power that previously did not exist—has been born in recent decades and is clearly making steady progress: initiatives targeted at resolving social issues that are initiated by NPOs, the business sector working through CSR activities, and so on. In Japan, for example, the Great East Japan Earthquake and tsunami disaster of 2011 has elevated people's conscious sense of social participation to unprecedented levels.

In Japan and 117 countries worldwide, the Nippon Foundation has abundant experience at the forefront of activities making social contributions.

Today my aspiration is to employ this vast experience and our far-reaching networks and make the Nippon Foundation a hub that sets "chemical reactions" to work in society, transcending individual positions so as to connect organizations, human resources, knowhow and funds.

In its second half-century, our goal is to make the Nippon Foundation a hub that will progressively enlarge the scope of social innovations, connecting people, organizations and activities to create a society in which all people will furnish support to one another. I believe the Foundation's very *raison d'être* rests in the advantages reaped from its involvement, the acceleration in speed we can provide in causing "chemical reactions" in society, and our ability to make new things happen.

3

INDIA, LAND OF "MOTHER GANGES"

India, Leprosy and Gandhi

India eliminates leprosy as a public health problem

For many years I have travelled the world on a mission to eliminate leprosy. One country I have focused on in particular is India, and in this chapter I look back over my activities there and discuss the current status of and future outlook for leprosy and people affected by the disease.

India is the second most populous nation on earth, its population currently tallying near 1.31 billion (as of 2017). A nation of numerous ethnic minorities, India uses Hindi and English as the official languages of government, and there are 22 officially recognized languages, of which Hindi is the most widely used. In addition, some two thousand local languages and dialects are in use. The dominant religion is Hinduism and the country is also home to Muslims, Christians, Sikhs, Buddhists and followers of other religious faiths. As a result, though it exists as one sovereign state, India might better be referred to as a diverse amalgamation of social and religious communities and groups.

India and Japan have a relationship dating back to antiquity. In ancient times India was known to Japan as the land that gave birth to Buddhism, giving it a special quality in the Japanese consciousness. In the Meiji period (1868–1912) exchanges between private citizens of the two countries flourished, as illustrated by the establishment of the Japan-India Association in 1903 by a distinguished group including Shigenobu Okuma (1838–1922) and Eiichi Shibusawa (1840–1931). Especially well known in Japan today are the close ties formed with Rash Behari Bose (1886–1945) and Subhas Chandra Bose (1897–1945), leaders of the Indian independence movement. In the postwar era Japan established diplomatic relations with India in 1952, and the friendly ties between the two countries have been maintained and further

99

developed through to the present day. India stands out as one of Japan's most faithful friends.

When I first started going to India, it accounted for the bulk of the world's new cases of leprosy. It is fair to say that India and leprosy were somehow linked in the popular imagination. It was a country where prejudice against leprosy and people affected by the disease ran deep. A variety of social and religious factors unique to India contributed to this bias, among them the country's stringent caste system, acute poverty and the inability of the educational system to reach all sectors of the vast population. It was believed in some quarters that leprosy is punishment for evil deeds performed in a previous life, so that once a person contracts it, he or she is quickly ostracized. As a result, even if someone sensed they might have the disease, they avoided treatment. A lack of proper knowledge about leprosy, including the misconception that the disease was incurable, also served to exacerbate the condition of patients who chose to conceal their affliction from society.

The idea that India would one day eliminate leprosy as a public health problem—bring the prevalence rate of the disease below 1 case per 10,000 people at the national level—seemed far-fetched. Yet with the implementation of multidrug therapy and other factors, this is what it proceeded to do, reducing prevalence from a level of nearly 58 per 10,000 of the population in 1983 to less than 1 by the end of 2005.

In January 2006 the Indian Government issued a formal announcement proclaiming that the target of eliminating leprosy as a public health problem, as defined by the WHO, had been achieved. Thanks to the determination and sustained efforts of everyone involved, the impossible had been accomplished—and accomplished much earlier than anyone predicted.

Reaching the elimination target in India was only one battle won in the greater war against leprosy, however. This huge country continues to account for around 60% of the world's new cases of leprosy. Nevertheless, the achievement gave those of us who had long worked toward that goal a significant boost of confidence: confident that if elimination as a public health problem was possible, then eradication may be so one day; and confident, too, that the human rights issues surrounding leprosy could definitely be resolved as well. Though the path would not be easy, it was a road down which we then, more than ever, were determined to proceed. This redoubling of our determination, of our confidence, was due entirely to this milestone that had been achieved by India.

The need to stay focused

Having achieved elimination at the national level, the next goal was to achieve elimination at the sub-national level. At time of writing, 34 out of India's 36 states and Union Territories have achieved a prevalence of less than 1 per 10,000, and 551 districts out of 669 had done so.

But to get to this point required further efforts on the part of many people. In the interim, I have made numerous visits to India and also met with Indian health officials on trips to the WHO headquarters in Geneva. It was necessary to keep people focused on leprosy, because there was a natural tendency in many countries to slacken off after the national elimination target had been reached.

At the WHO General Assembly in Geneva in May 2011, for example, I conveyed my concerns about states and districts that had yet to achieve elimination to the Deputy Minister of India's Ministry of Health and Family Welfare, and we discussed what might be done. After listening intently to my views, the Deputy Minister immediately determined to convene a meeting to discuss the issues raised, to be attended by the Deputy Health Ministers of the states where the elimination target had yet to be reached. Thanks to his decisive action and swift resolve, the meeting took place two and a half months later, in August, in Delhi.

In attendance, besides the Deputy Minister who had arranged the event, were an array of other officials from the Ministry of Health and Family Welfare, 14 representatives from the 13 states where leprosy remained a concern, representatives of the WHO Country Office for India, and numerous specialists.

A measure was proposed calling for district leprosy officers to be posted to every district. Meanwhile, deep concern was also expressed over the fact that 1 of every 10 patients in India was a child, prompting discussions on the need to adopt special measures for coping with this segment of the population.

Discussions also focused on the need to pursue early detection and treatment of patients in regions that had yet to achieve the elimination target, with specific approaches to be drawn up based on the special characteristics and current status of each state.

The official in charge of Delhi, for example, pointed out that 50% of leprosy patients in the state were internal migrants from other states, a fact that made it difficult to acquire an accurate overview of the number of patients in Delhi. The delegate from Orissa (now Odisha) described how leprosy was rife among the tribal groups living in remote locations. He discussed how a system of health assistants had been established at the grass-roots level to locate new patients, as well as giving an overview of how the assistants were trained. Early detection and early treatment of new patients are the best means of preventing the physical deformities that become the main cause of discrimination against persons who contract this disease.

Mahatma Gandhi, my spiritual father

The first time I visited India in conjunction with leprosy-related activities was in February 1984, when I attended the 12th International Leprosy Congress in New Delhi. Indira Gandhi (1917–1984) and Mother Teresa (1910–1997) were among the participants on that occasion. Subsequently, as a result of the WHO's 2nd and 6th International Conferences on Leprosy Elimination (1995 and 1999, respectively), I began making frequent visits to India. Over the years I have now visited the country more than fifty times, including short stays of three or four days. Some years I visit as many as seven times.

If I dare say so myself, I am amazed at this continuing schedule of visits. I imagine few of my fellow countrymen have visited India as much as I have.

Helping India to eliminate leprosy as a public health problem was something I had been keen to achieve. Today one of my biggest goals in life is to continue my involvement in India, and do what I can to support the country in its ongoing efforts to achieve leprosy-free status one day.

Today India is like a second homeland to me. My activities there have presented me with a host of difficult challenges and hardships. At the same time, to the extent that I have struggled to overcome these, India has also given me consummate joy. In a sense, India has instilled in me a deep appreciation of life even more than Japan, the country of my birth.

Whenever I undertake my activities in India, an image that I always have uppermost in mind is that of Mahatma Gandhi (1869–1948). Gandhi, considered the father of the Indian independence movement, devoted himself in no small way to the care of leprosy patients.

Gandhi was a member of India's elite. Born the son of a *diwan*, a chief minister of state, he studied law and became a barrister. In mid-career, however, he chose to shed his position of privilege and wealth and began preaching the power of nonviolence and disobedience. He carried out what he preached, winning the release of his fellow countrymen from the yoke of British rule. He also fought to eliminate various forms of discrimination, such as discrimination based on race, gender, economic status, religion and social class. Rabindranath Tagore (1861–1941), the famed poet and a close friend of Gandhi, referred to him as "the embodiment of courage and sacrifice".

There is a well-known anecdote about Gandhi concerning leprosy. Invited to open a leprosy hospital, he said that opening a hospital was something ordinary, but that he would come to close it one day.

Unfortunately Gandhi did not get to keep his pledge: on 30 January 1948 he was assassinated in New Delhi by a Hindu fundamentalist. Today, 30 January is designated as Anti-Leprosy Day to keep alive the memory of Gandhi's selfless efforts to care for people affected by leprosy—he once stated that if India has the breath of life in it, it must stop turning its back on people with leprosy.

In December 2003 I had the unforgettable experience of visiting the Sevagram Ashram in the Wardha district of Maharashtra state, in central India. This is where Gandhi created a residence that became a centre of his activities, and as someone who is deeply involved in efforts to eliminate leprosy, I had long wished to visit this place so closely tied to Gandhi's life.

The ashram was swept immaculately clean and was a haven of tranquillity. A huge sal tree provided a welcome cover of shade. Gandhi stayed here on numerous occasions starting in 1936, using it as a place of meditation. It is also said that it was here that he treated a friend who had leprosy. Today Sevagram Ashram is preserved in its original state as a historical landmark.

The buildings at the ashram are all of extremely modest construction, earthen tiled roofs capping simple mud walls. Gandhi's room is bare except for a bed and spinning wheel—and, incongruously, a telephone booth. I heard that the phone was installed by the colonial authorities so that they could keep in touch with Gandhi for consultations, but he used it to communicate with his freedom fighters working for independence. In this way, Gandhi's quiet retreat also served as a base for patriots burning with the aspiration to win India's freedom from British rule.

One step through the ashram gate takes the visitor immediately back into the hubbub so characteristic of India. A cacophony of vehicles streams by, the destitute of all ages flock around, and the city streets, filled with noise, extend on toward the horizon. To think of Gandhi's vision, seeing the future of India rising above this chaotic scene, moved me deeply.

My father, who led me down the path of leprosy work, hated leprosy from the bottom of his heart as a disease that takes human beings no different from any other and plunges them into a state of despair. He pledged to rid the world of this cruel disease, and for more than forty years he energetically worked to carry out his mission. Death took him, however, before his life's goal was achieved.

The image of my father, a man who worked selflessly without any self-interest, overlaps in my mind with Gandhi, a man who dedicated his life to win India its freedom, to help the multitudes of oppressed, and to ease the suffering of those afflicted with leprosy.

Ryoichi Sasakawa and Mahatma Gandhi. These two mortals, now gone, are both beloved "fathers" who continuously guide me down the path I was meant to follow, lighting my way steadily like the Pole Star pointing north.

Persons Affected by Leprosy in Leading Roles

What I have done in India

My approach to helping India eliminate leprosy as a public health problem can be summarized in the following six points: establish a target; remain firmly determined to achieve full success; visit in person; confirm results with my own eyes; meet with people in the highest positions and request their understanding and cooperation; and maintain good relationships with the media and seek their cooperation.

The ultimate target was clear from the outset: to rid India of both leprosy and the discrimination the disease causes. I then asked myself what form of cooperation would be best in order to achieve that target in the least amount of time. The answer I landed on was to personally meet with people affected by leprosy, to talk with them, and hear their wants. Based on these, I and the people working with me would immediately set out to do what we could.

There are some things that I, as an ordinary citizen, am incapable of doing, so I focused on using my position and networks to take my message to those in high positions in government, seeking their understanding and cooperation. To spread correct knowledge about leprosy, communication with the media would also be indispensable.

Concerning results of the various activities that would be undertaken, instead of glancing through reports and taking what they might say at face value, I would invariably confirm the results for myself.

And so each task would begin with hearing the wants of people affected by leprosy; and each task would end with my checking all outcomes for myself. In this way, by repeating this process again and again I found myself with increasing opportunities to visit India.

Empowering persons affected by leprosy

Toward the end of 2005, as India drew closer to eliminating leprosy as a public health problem at the national level, I felt that efforts to eliminate social discrimination were lagging behind. Travelling the length and breadth of India, this was my honest impression at the time.

To tackle the issue of discrimination, I felt a new approach was needed. The public needed to see persons affected by leprosy as ordinary human beings no different from themselves. If there could be opportunities for persons affected to make their voices heard, despite the courage it would take to speak out in the face of the prejudice they faced and tell their stories, I felt this would make a difference. Convinced that persons affected by leprosy must be the agents of change in rooting out the prejudice toward the disease in India, I determined to redouble my efforts in India with this strategy in mind.

On 27 January 2005 I visited Gandhi Smriti in New Delhi, a museum located in the house where Mahatma Gandhi had been residing when, on 30 January, 1948, he was felled by three gunshots fired by a Hindu fundamentalist. It is said that Gandhi was walking in the garden after dinner on his way to offer evening prayers when the shots rang out. Without making a sound he collapsed to the ground, placing one hand to his forehead in a gesture of forgiveness to the assassin. According to some accounts, his final words were "Rama, Rama", a call to his most beloved god.

I slowly walked along the same path Gandhi had taken. Thinking of the quiet way he had ended his life, as though he had had a premonition of its coming, I headed to a rally that had been scheduled here at the museum to mark the starting point of the new battle to eliminate discrimination against leprosy.

The rally had been organized at the suggestion of Dr. S.D. Gokhale (1925–2013), president of the International Leprosy Union (ILU), and its purpose was not to undertake specialized discussions concerning leprosy in keeping with convention, but rather to seek cooperation from the media and from persons affected with leprosy in conducting elimination activities.

The gathering opened with words of welcome offered by India's former President Ramaswamy Venkataraman (1910–2009). He was followed by a succession of people—the WHO representative to India, for example—at the vanguard of elimination activities, all voicing determination to complete the task ahead and pledging strong support for the efforts of everyone involved in eradicating leprosy as well as the social discrimination toward this disease.

The atmosphere, filled with a unified sense of purpose and ebullient determination, was befitting this gathering convening at a place so closely associated with Mahatma Gandhi. It seemed like a gift given by Gandhi himself.

Among the two hundred participants, more than two-thirds—134 in all—were persons affected by leprosy from nine of India's states. In Indian society, identifying oneself as a person affected by leprosy is in itself an extremely painful act. But the people who participated that day had all been cured of their disease and, with great courage, had rejoined society and proceeded to work actively in their respective occupations. These participants were sustained by their own achievements and self-confidence, and they eagerly offered their cooperation in conducting media campaigns of enlightenment in the regions where they lived and worked.

The rally also served as an occasion for appointing 32 activists among the participating persons affected by leprosy as "lokdoots" (ambassadors) representing all those in situations similar to theirs. Their appointment was decided as a way to give visibility to the role of persons affected by leprosy as central figures in activities that target the disease's elimination.

The people affected by leprosy who attended the rally, especially those who were appointed to serve as ambassadors, would, I felt sure, contribute greatly to raising awareness in their regions. My role, I took to heart, would be to provide my all-round support to their activities and to create a framework that would enable the scope of their activities to steadily expand.

Gathering strength from persons affected by leprosy: Pune, March 2005

Pune is the second-largest city, after Mumbai, in India's Maharashtra state, which has a population of roughly 100 million. A conference was held here in March 2005 on matters pertaining to leprosy-related human rights and discrimination. I participated together with Professor Yozo Yokota of Chuo University. Professor Yokota was to submit a report of a study on leprosy and human rights issues to the upcoming meeting of the UN Sub-Commission on the Promotion and Protection of Human Rights, and he had already attended meetings and seminars in Africa and Brazil, collecting information and meeting with people involved in these matters.

The conference was jointly organized by the Nippon Foundation, the Sasakawa Memorial Health Foundation, the International Leprosy Union, and the India chapter of IDEA, the International Association for Integration, Dignity and Economic Advancement, an organization of and for persons affected by leprosy. In addition to leprosy specialists, it was attended by representatives from the legal profession, NGOs, human rights groups and others as well as persons affected by leprosy. Opinions were exchanged on a broad range of topics from health services, education, residence, marriage, families, inheritance and disability prevention to social isolation, stigma and legal matters.

As the conference got under way, one of the participants asked why it had been decided to take up the issue of leprosy-related human rights at this point in time. "To be frank, we were completely ignorant," responded Professor Yokota. "At the UN no recognition had been made of the fact that human rights issues of this scale exist in contemporary society." I was deeply moved by the candour of the professor's response.

In India, 11 million people had already been cured thanks to MDT, and yet even as of 2005 there still existed numerous isolation colonies, and their very presence attests to the discrimination, misunderstanding and prejudice that still exist in Indian society. It was still common to refer to people as "lepers" or "leprosy patients" even after they had been cured of the disease. Professor Yokota's admission of total ignorance with respect to the human rights dimension of leprosy had, with brilliant succinctness, got to the core of the issue that needed to be addressed. For all the years I had been focused on eliminating the disease of leprosy, I was suddenly made to realize, and sorely regret, that my own attention to this aspect of the leprosy issue had been inadequate, too.

That said, I also felt that India had been changing, gradually. As the example of Dr. Gopal, the IDEA India president, demonstrated, an increasing number of people affected by leprosy were being accepted by society and were beginning to raise their voices. Dr. Gopal became a model of hope for Indians affected by leprosy, as I have described in Chapter 1.

"Until now persons affected by leprosy didn't consider the discrimination rooted in prejudice that was directed against them as a violation of their human rights," Dr. Gopal once told me. "They merely reconciled themselves to such discrimination as a matter of fate."

Among those who had recovered from their disease, some bemoaned the fact that when they had contracted leprosy, they went from being a member of a certain caste to being a member of the caste known as "leprosy". Now, however, people affected by leprosy were finally breaking their silence and beginning to voice their opinions. Conferences and meetings led by people affected by leprosy had also begun increasing in number. The time had arrived when they were beginning to get involved in activities to eliminate this disease.

After this conference on leprosy-related human rights, I moved to New Delhi and had an audience with Prime Minister Manmohan Singh. The Prime Minister was very familiar with the situation surrounding leprosy in his country and with our activities to eliminate the disease. "You are doing noble work," he said to me. "You have been an inspiration to India." When I told Mr. Singh about our three messages—that leprosy is a curable disease, that medicine is available free of charge, and that discrimination against leprosy is unacceptable—he repeated them over and over to himself, and then gave me his pledge to do everything he could to eliminate leprosy in India and improve the human rights of those affected.

Sowing the seeds of a network of persons affected by leprosy: Kolkata and Chennai, May 2005

In May 2005 conferences on the elimination of leprosy were convened in Kolkata (formerly Calcutta) and Chennai (formerly Madras). Kolkata is located in West Bengal, a state in India's north-east that borders on Bhutan to the north, Bangladesh to the east, and Nepal to the north-west. Kolkata, the state capital, is India's third-largest city after Mumbai and Delhi, famed as the birthplace of Tagore and the home of Mother Teresa's Missionaries of Charity.

The conference here had been organized by the International Leprosy Union, with backing from the Nippon Foundation. Its theme was advocacy strategy and the role of the media in eliminating leprosy. Dr. S.D. Gokhale, the ILU president, gave a powerful presentation on the social circumstances surrounding leprosy. "If society won't change," he averred, "then we have to change society."

While I attended the meeting, I received pledges of solid support from West Bengal's Chief Minister, Buddhadeb Bhattacharjee, and from its Minister of Health and Family Welfare, Dr. Surjya Kanta Misra. Chief Minister Bhattacharjee demonstrated a profound understanding of the problems surrounding leprosy, and he pointed to two critical issues in particular: enhancing popular understanding and improving social rehabilitation.

Chennai, the capital of Tamil Nadu, India's southernmost state, is situated on the country's eastern coast facing the Bay of Bengal. Until 1996 the city, India's third most populous, was known as Madras, the name given to it during British colonial times. The eastern coast of India—the second-longest sea coast in the world—was the scene of a significant number of casualties during the devastating tsunami triggered by the Indian Ocean earthquake of December 2004.

The Regional Conference on Leprosy held in Chennai in May 2005 was co-hosted by IDEA India, the Leprosy Elimination Alliance and the Indian Leprosy Association (Hind Kusht Nivaran Sangh). The conference drew participants from the four states of southern India where leprosy had earlier been most prevalent: Kerala, Karnataka, Andhra Pradesh and Tamil Nadu, including representatives of government, the medical field, people affected by leprosy, NGO representatives and members of the legal profession. All four of those states have now succeeded in reaching the elimination target.

Of particular interest were reports presented by jurists who specialize in human rights issues. They pointed out how many laws in India were problematic from a human rights perspective, citing provisions such as those restricting persons affected by leprosy from accessing public spaces, and others making leprosy grounds for divorce.

A film of considerable relevance was introduced at the conference. Known in English as *Blood Tears*, the film *Raktha Kanneeru* was a 2003 remake of a Tamil film originally released in 1954, and its storyline aroused much debate. The main character in the film has dalliances with numerous women, and as "divine punishment" for his misdeeds he contracts leprosy. The film was introduced at the conference to illustrate the false notions too often propagated by the media. India has an enormous number of film enthusiasts, and the influence wielded by the film industry in fuelling unfounded prejudice of this kind needs to be recognized and dealt with.

In tandem with attending the conference in Chennai, I paid a visit to the Villivakkam Leprosy Colony located in a low-income district in the northern quarters of the city. My visit coincided with a monthly meeting of leaders of leprosy colonies in Tamil Nadu. At one time Tamil Nadu had the most leprosy patients of any region in India, and there are close to seventy colonies in the state. A state-wide network of people affected by leprosy had already been formed, and it was working with dedication to improve the quality of life in the colonies.

One example of the achievements made at the Villivakkam Leprosy Colony is the presence of a labour and delivery room within the colony's clinic that is open to residents of the surrounding community. This enables 110 families living inside the colony to mix with the neighbouring community, a situation that has broken down the barriers between the colony and the "outside" world.

Inspired by what I saw at Villivakkam, I proposed convening a nationwide meeting of leaders from all leprosy colonies throughout India. My proposal was favourably received by the entire body of core members attending the Chennai regional conference.

In order to bring such a conference to fruition, I recognized the need first to undertake an investigation into the current situation of the numerous leprosy colonies said to exist in the country.

Leprosy colonies were generally formed by persons affected by leprosy as a response to being ostracized by their own communities. This circumstance made it extremely difficult to get an accurate understanding of how many colonies were in existence, where they were, and how large they were, a difficulty

109

compounded by the fact that India had no comprehensive statistical material offering such information. Before leaders of the leprosy colonies nationwide could be assembled, it was therefore essential to gather information on the colonies that actually existed. Dr. Gopal generously agreed to undertake this investigation, with support provided by the Nippon Foundation.

One other thing necessary was the creation of a new network connecting people affected by leprosy with the media, NGOs and industry. Were this to be realized, it would surely be the first in India, if not the world. In the meantime, there needed to be an organization of and for people affected by leprosy, as I felt sure this would advance the movement for the elimination of the disease and the discrimination associated with it.

Bringing the media on the team: Media Partnership Workshops, 2005

In September and October 2005, in my position as the WHO Goodwill Ambassador for Leprosy Elimination I participated in Media Partnership Workshops at four locations: Kolkata (West Bengal), Patna (Bihar), Guwahati (Assam) and Lucknow (Uttar Pradesh). The four states where the workshops were held had all previously suffered from high prevalence rates, but progress had steadily been made that had a positive impact on eliminating the disease as a public health problem throughout India. Nevertheless, while the target prevalence rates may have been achieved, the social rehabilitation of people affected by leprosy remained a challenge.

Media Partnership Workshops were convened a total of eight times, organized by the ILU with cooperation from a private communications consultancy. The objective of the first four workshops, held in September and October, was to provide correct knowledge about leprosy to members of the major media associations, to seek their cooperation in eliminating prejudice and discrimination, and, through their reporting, to help eliminate leprosy and resolve the human rights issues surrounding this affliction.

In all, approximately 150 members of the media attended the day-long workshops in the four states, considerably more than we had anticipated. We found, however, that they had virtually no knowledge whatsoever concerning leprosy. The workshops were also attended by the various state governors, state health ministers and WHO representatives, who took turns addressing the media members on the importance of awareness building and asked for their cooperation. Also attending each of the workshops were some twenty to thirty students aspiring to become journalists in their respective regions. Their participation, as members of the younger generation, was invited as a way of eliminating discrimination against leprosy long into the future.

There is a common perception that as progress is made in eliminating leprosy and the number of patients steadily declines, the number of people subjected to discrimination will also decline. But while the number of individuals who suffer discrimination may indeed grow smaller, there can be no fundamental solution to the problem of social discrimination unless the number of people who discriminate against people affected by the disease also diminishes. This is a point that often tends to get overlooked, and to reduce the number of people who engage in discrimination it is necessary to change social awareness—and to do so, initiatives to spread correct knowledge about leprosy are absolutely essential.

I had always felt that one reason prejudice and discrimination toward leprosy had long been able to persist on a global scale was because of the way the media covered leprosy. In their quest to attract the attention of their readers or viewers, the media had often engaged in sensational reporting, without confirming the accuracy of their information and ignoring the privacy and rights of persons affected by leprosy. When those who work in the media themselves have incorrect knowledge about the disease and report in ways that exacerbate the social stigma against persons affected by leprosy, one cannot expect those on the receiving end of such information, who are inevitably susceptible to accepting what the media tells them as fact, to realize where the real truth is to be found.

India of course was no exception to this prevailing trend. I strongly hoped that through participation in a Media Partnership Workshop some media members, even if only a few in number, would come to seriously address issues surrounding leprosy in their reporting.

Particularly in so far as leprosy is concerned, from my experience working with local media I know that we who convey the messages about this disease have to be more strategic in how we provide news and stories to the media. Regrettably, the topic of leprosy elimination tends to be thought of as having little news value, so it is accorded low priority by the media. If we seek for the media to be more proactive in their reporting on leprosy, then we who provide information to them must create mechanisms that will enable such information to be provided smoothly.

At the Media Partnership Workshops, news and TV reporters and editors were given briefings about leprosy, shown a documentary about leprosy and human rights, and presented with a book, written in the Hindi and Bengali languages, titled *Dignity Regained*, relating the personal experiences of 12 people affected by leprosy. Through the workshops we wanted the participants to comprehend the misery suffered by people affected by leprosy because of the discrimination directed toward them, to recognize the efforts they make every day to reintegrate themselves into society, and to realize that people affected by leprosy are no different from normal healthy people: they are all vibrant individuals each unique in his or her own way.

If, through participation in workshops, more and more members of the media turn their attention to the lives and experiences of people affected by leprosy, we could expect an increase in proper reporting that respects the latter's dignity as human beings and their individuality. Then, if the number of people who see or hear such reports increases, gradually we should be able to dispel the prejudice and discrimination that associate leprosy with "filth," poverty" and "divine punishment".

As I travelled about the four states where the workshops were held, I eagerly welcomed interviews by the media and responded to a wide variety of their questions. On some days I was individually interviewed by as many as 12 newspapers, and I appeared on TV as well. The questions I was asked were nearly identical every time: overwhelmingly, they concerned how leprosy is transmitted and leprosy's infection rate. Even after participating in a workshop and gaining an intellectual understanding of the information provided to them, in reality they still remained fearful of leprosy. Some media members could be found making unconscious use of discriminatory terms, "leper" being a common example.

Changing people's perceptions is no easy matter. No information, no matter how correct, is internalized by its recipient on first encounter. The only effective means of winning a true understanding and acceptance of information is by conveying it over and over again, hundreds or thousands of time, like a tape recorder.

In that respect it was very significant that the workshops were also attended by many young people aspiring to become journalists. A contest was even held to create posters on the topic of "leprosy elimination". The call for entries had been issued in advance, and the works submitted were judged during the workshop. The three "best" teams were presented with awards.

Among the entries, a large number depicted persons with leprosy in a tragic light, offering the message that "because they are so pitiful, we should extend them a helping hand". As I said, the posters were created before the workshop, and I was eager to know whether after participating in the workshop the impressions toward leprosy of the students who made them had changed, so I asked the students who won the contest about this. They said their notions about people affected by leprosy had changed after gaining proper knowledge about the disease.

Through this experiment I came to realize the importance of taking up a positive image of leprosy embodied in my three core messages within school curriculums, as I now felt that doing so would offer favourable possibilities. If the younger generation, who are not rigid in their thinking, are given the right information, then with the gradual change of generations I am convinced that the perception will spread of leprosy as a "disease that is not frightening", giving increased impetus to the resolution of the problems of discrimination and prejudice and, ultimately, to the realization of a society free of discrimination.

Birth of the National Forum, Achievement of Elimination in India

Nationwide conference of people affected by leprosy, December 2005

19 December 2005 was a day that became one of the most memorable of my lifetime. It was on this date that a nationwide gathering of persons affected by leprosy—India's first ever—took place in Delhi. Dubbed the National Forum, the event launched a call, by the very people who were affected by leprosy, for the elimination of discrimination and restoration of their dignity.

The meeting was organized by the Leprosy Colony Project Secretariat, with support from the Nippon Foundation and the Sasakawa Memorial Health Foundation.

Bringing together persons affected by leprosy who represented their respective colonies, having them share their knowledge and experiences, and providing them with an opportunity to begin raising their voices, in unity, to Indian society constituted an important stepping stone toward subsequent action. Linking together the leprosy colonies scattered throughout the country and undertaking activities to eliminate prejudice and discrimination toward leprosy on a national scale would surely succeed in changing society

The Federation of Indian Chambers of Commerce and Industry (FICCI) Golden Jubilee Auditorium, where the conference took place, was filled to capacity with 580 participants, and the atmosphere was electric with excitement even before the proceedings began. Included among those present were 450 people affected by leprosy who had gathered from all across India. The majority had never travelled by railway or aeroplane before. Many had been subjected to severe discrimination because of their disease, forced to leave their homes and live in colonies. Even after they had been cured, they remained without means of livelihood and eked out an existence by begging. Many of these people were travelling to Delhi for the first time in their lives to attend this conference.

Staying in a hotel was also a new experience for many of them, and they appeared especially thrilled to be able to lodge this way just as "normal" people do. With great excitement they told me of their joy at sleeping in a comfortable bed with fresh white sheets, or washing their bodies with hot water.

Originally the participants had been booked to stay at the YMCA and a deposit had been paid. But when the YMCA learned that the scheduled guests were people affected by leprosy, the reservation had been cancelled. Next, a request was made to stay at a state-owned hotel. One stroke of good fortune was that the person working for the National Office of Tourism was Leena Nandan, a woman who had previously worked vigorously to help eliminate leprosy as a project director for the National Leprosy Elimination Programme in Uttar Pradesh. Thanks to her, the hotel, after some initial hesitation, agreed to provide the people affected by leprosy with exactly the same services as its "regular" guests.

Dr. Gopal, in his position as president of IDEA India, had cooperated with the Nippon Foundation in conducting a fact-finding survey of leprosy colonies in India, according to which a total of 630 colonies had been confirmed in 23 of the country's 35 states and territories as of December 2004. (Subsequent surveys have confirmed some 850 colonies to date.) The survey also revealed that all colonies had leaders, and many of them were in Delhi to attend this conference.

A key event that emerged from the conference was the adoption of what is known as the Delhi Declaration of Dignity. The declaration was read to the assembled audience by Nevis Mary, an Indian woman, then 47, who had contracted leprosy when she was 20. Not long after the nature of her illness became known to her and her family, her father succumbed from the shock while Nevis herself suffered severe discrimination both at school and, later, at her workplace. Today, she is happily married to a very understanding and supportive husband, and to help those who have had the same sorrowful experience, she has vigorously taken up the cause and is active in seeking the elimination of discrimination against people affected by leprosy.

Ms. Mary read the declaration expressing the determination of persons affected by leprosy to join forces in seeking restoration of their personal dignity and fundamental human rights—in a strong voice filled with confidence. The audience responded with rapturous applause.

The participants at the conference, both people affected by leprosy and individuals working to support the cause of leprosy, proceeded to discuss a variety of topics necessary for their campaign to advance to the next step. With great zeal they exchanged views on how to move forward, and out of these discussions it was decided that the conference should be convened on a regular basis and a National Forum office created. Specific action plans were also drawn up.

One participant affected by leprosy, a gentleman of small stature who always wore a white suit and necktie, proposed that use of the term "leprosy" itself, with its ingrained negative overtones, should be eliminated. For many years he had battled vigorously against the authorities to improve the lot of leprosy sufferers, and recalling the discrimination he himself had endured, he addressed the assembly. "I don't think of myself as a weak person," he proclaimed. "If something needs to be accomplished, then it must be achieved not by others but by one's own hands. For this, it's necessary to gain self-confidence in one's own strength; otherwise the battle cannot be won."

Another participant, the leader of a colony in Haryana state close to Delhi, spoke of his own experience. "Twenty to thirty years ago I was a beggar and I never imagined I would be speaking at a large conference like this," he said with great emotion. "Now that momentum to change things is growing among people affected by leprosy, we should hold meetings all around the country, even in small villages, to spread the word further and change the common perception toward leprosy."

As these speakers declared, now that the "light" had been lit, it should never be allowed to be extinguished. To ensure that the momentum did not cease with the completion of the survey of colonies and the close of the conference at hand, I was convinced that meetings of this kind must continue and the passion and determination shown by its participants must be carried forward. With emotion rising inside me, holding back my tears, I addressed the assembly: "I will continue to walk side by side with you, offering my full support. You have my promise."

Two participants were on hand from the Indian Government: Union Minister of Social Justice and Empowerment, Meira Kumar, and Union Minister of State for Statistics and Programme Implementation, Oscar Fernandes. Ms. Kumar spoke of her involvement in eliminating discrimination by revising her nation's divorce laws and by securing a 3% quota for educational and employment opportunities for the disabled, including people affected by leprosy. Mr. Fernandes pledged to listen to the voices of people affected by leprosy, his fellow countrymen and women, and to do everything he could to remove the lingering stigma against them.

As the conference drew to its end, one of the participants, an elderly woman from Haryana, approached me with a look of great joy in her eyes. "I was late in arriving and didn't receive the bag and shawl that were given to all the delegates," she began. "But what I got here today was something I had never received in the forty years since I contracted leprosy: respect and dignity." Watching her leave the hall, with a spring in her step, I was overcome with the renewed conviction that a great step forward had been taken in the fight to eliminate leprosy, and the stigma attached to it, in India.

I also felt certain that 19 December 2005 would go down in history as the first time people affected by leprosy had spoken out in public on such a scale, and that the events of that day would mark a new beginning for their activities.

Immediately after the conference, news emerged that India had achieved the goal of eliminating leprosy as a public health problem.

Not wanting to let this golden opportunity pass, and to give a further boost to people affected by leprosy in their quest to be accepted by society, I launched the first Global Appeal to End Stigma and Discrimination against People Affected by Leprosy at the India Habitat Centre in New Delhi. The event took place on 29 January 2006; it was the last Sunday of the month, the day designated as World Leprosy Day. In response to my call for support, the Global Appeal was endorsed by eleven prominent leaders from around the world, including five Nobel Peace Prize Laureates—former U.S. President Jimmy Carter, His Holiness the 14th Dalai Lama, Archbishop Desmond Tutu, Oscar Arias and Elie Wiesel—and the President of Brazil, Luiz Inácio Lula da Silva.

In various ways the path to self-reliance of people affected by leprosy is impeded by discrimination. For those who have the desire and the capacity to work, nothing is more cruel than being forced to live out their lives robbed of employment opportunities. If only they are given opportunities to study and to work, people affected by leprosy should be able to manifest their ability to function as productive members of society, no different from everyone else.

The Global Appeal programme was organized, at my suggestion, by the Nippon Foundation to inform the world of the reality of the situation of people affected by leprosy and thereby persuade people everywhere to extend a hand in support. I was certain that if I could get world leaders to endorse the Global Appeal and express their determination to join the fight against prejudice and discrimination toward leprosy, then society's perceptions of the disease would undergo a dramatic transformation.

Also in attendance at the India Habitat Centre that day were former Chief Justice of India Y.V. Chandrachud (1920–2008), International Leprosy Union president Dr. S.D. Gokhale (1925–2013), who had long devoted himself to.

our activities in India, Professor Yozo Yokota of Chuo University, special rapporteur on leprosy and human rights for the UN Sub-Commission on the Promotion and Protection of Human Rights, IDEA president Dr. P.K. Gopal, and many others who had served on the front lines in the fight against leprosy and its stigma. Representatives of people affected by leprosy also participated from Indonesia, the Philippines and Nepal, and together with their Indian counterparts they presented reports on the social discrimination they and their families experienced in their respective countries.

The following day we shifted our venue to Kolkata, capital of West Bengal state, and here, in the presence of the city's mayor and the state Minister of Justice, through the local media we again announced the Global Appeal. The Minister of Justice cited "correct awareness" as the most important factor enabling the elimination of discrimination and stigma against leprosy—a statement that struck a fresh new chord.

The same day, the Indian government issued its announcement that it had eliminated leprosy as a public health problem. India was the country with the largest number of people affected by leprosy in the world. The announcement that it had achieved the elimination target was thus especially momentous, as it marked an important step forward toward achieving the dream of a leprosy-free India embraced by both Mahatma Gandhi and Mother Teresa, and by my father Ryoichi Sasakawa, by me, by the Nippon Foundation and so many others. In this way, 30 January 2006 was a day on which the fight against leprosy shifted to a new stage.

The Quest for Self-reliance of People Affected by Leprosy

Sasakawa-India Leprosy Foundation

At the ceremony announcing the Global Appeal, I also announced a plan to raise funds in Japan and India and launch a mechanism, in the form of a foundation, to support the self-reliance of people affected by leprosy in India. This plan led to the establishment of the Sasakawa-India Leprosy Foundation (S-ILF).

S-ILF was inaugurated with three overarching aims: to create vocational training venues for people affected by leprosy, and to secure employment opportunities with cooperation from India's business community; to launch a microfinance programme under which persons affected by leprosy in need—especially women and families—can acquire such skills as embroidery and handiwork to enable them to secure a livelihood; and to create opportunities for education for children from leprosy-affected families by means of a scholarship programme.

I had always felt strongly the need for mechanisms of these kinds in order that people affected by leprosy might live independently without having to resort to begging. To establish S-ILF, the Nippon Foundation initially provided US$10 million in funding; but going forward it would also be necessary to seek cooperation from India's business sector and NGOs in raising funds to keep S-ILF in operation.

I thus proceeded to visit India a number of times, both to undertake the legal procedures necessary for setting up a foundation in that country and to meet with key members of India's business community, to ask for their understanding and support in raising funds for S-ILF's establishment. I paid visits to organizations such as the Confederation of Indian Industry (CII) and the Indian Chamber of Commerce (ICC), and I also arranged for group meetings with leaders from the country's economic sphere, academia and media, where I spoke to them on our objectives in creating S-ILF.

As a result of these initiatives, S-ILF was officially inaugurated in November 2006. The position of chairperson was filled by Dr. S.K. Noordeen, who for many years had been in charge of leprosy-related matters at the WHO and who at this time was serving as president of the International Leprosy Association. We also were fortunate to welcome on board Tarun Das, a core member of India's business community, in the position of trustee. To perform the day-to-day administration of S-ILF, we requested the cooperation of Dr. Vineeta Shanker, a prominent sociologist who enthusiastically endorsed S-ILF's founding objectives.

The decision to include "Sasakawa" in the name of the foundation was made based on a variety of considerations. In considering a name that would be most effective from the perspective of attracting funds, I believed that the greatest impact would be achieved by using my own surname, which, as a result of visiting India some twenty times over the preceding three years and carrying out my activities throughout the country, had already acquired a considerable level of recognition through the press and television. Affixing the name of an individual to a foundation this way is by no means unusual outside Japan, but within Japan doing so often arouses criticism of crossing the boundary between personal and public interests. The possibility of generating such criticism was of concern to me, but ultimately I determined to use my name in order to make the foundation as effective as possible.

On 26 March 2007 S-ILF convened its very first Board of Trustees meeting in Delhi. Discussions focused on the directions the foundation's activities

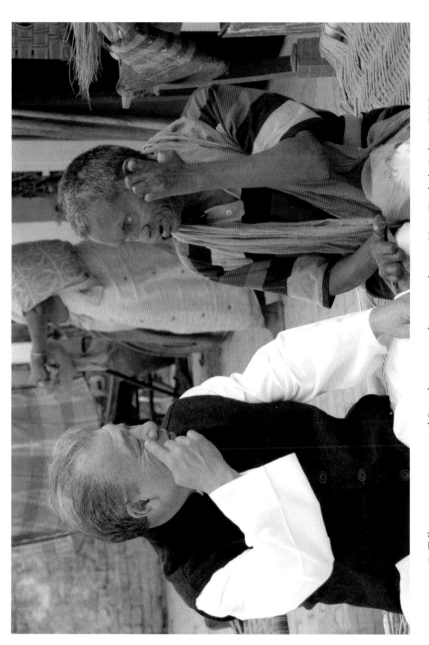

1. Talking to a person cured from leprosy at a leprosy colony in Uttar Pradesh, India in 2009.

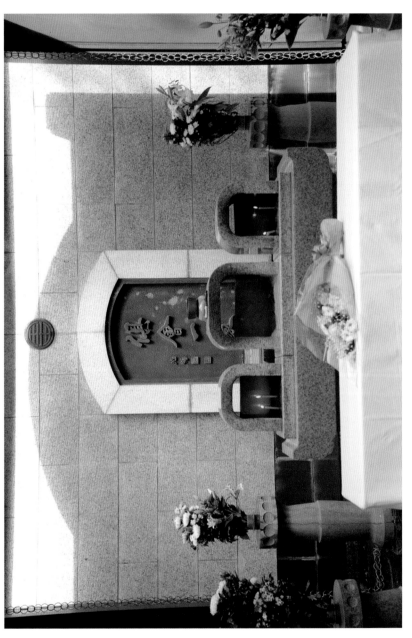

2. A crypt of the residents of the National Sanatorium Tama Zensho-en in Japan, who were insulated from their own families.

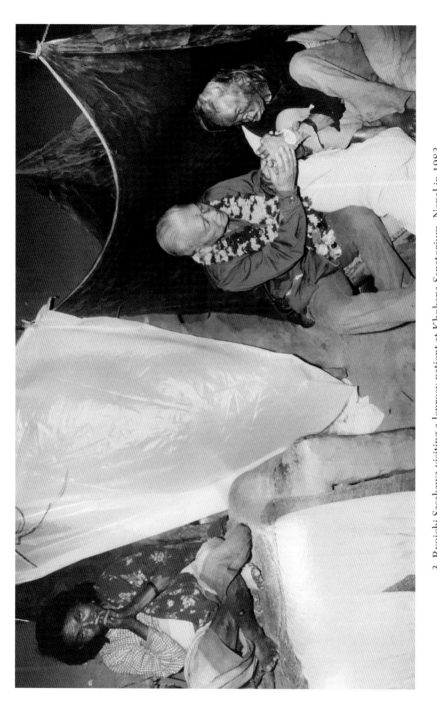

3. Ryoichi Sasakawa visiting a leprosy patient at Khokana Sanatorium, Nepal in 1983.

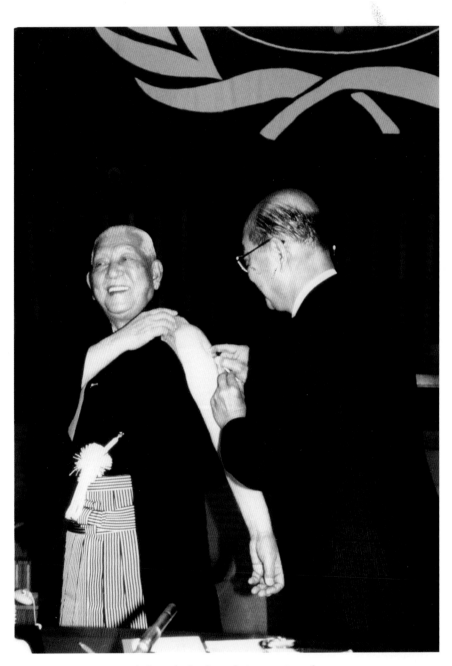

4. Ryoichi Sasakawa being vaccinated.

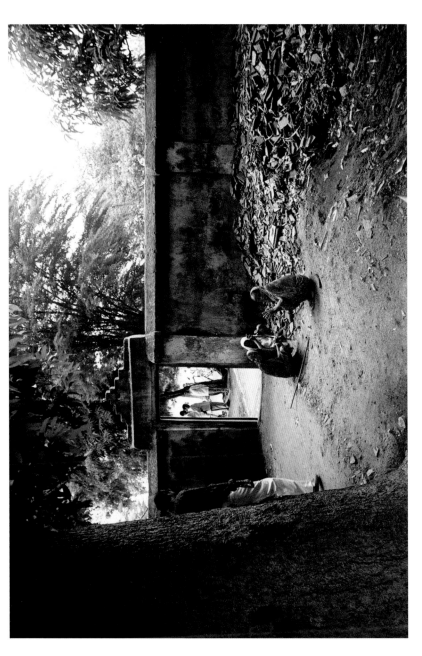

5. A wall symbolizes the isolation at the entrance of the residential area for persons affected by leprosy in Odisha, India in 2003.

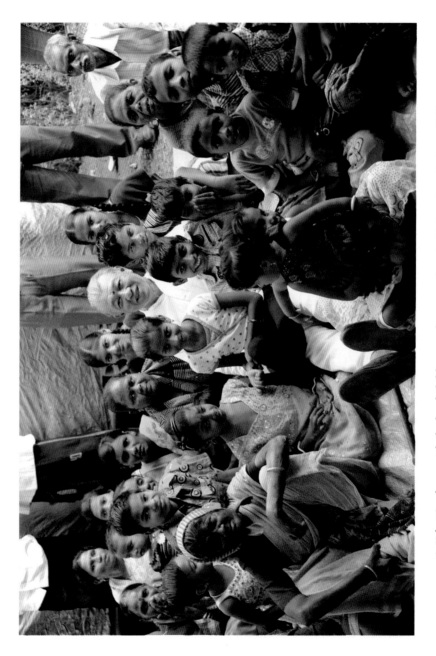

6. Yohei Sasakawa with the local children at a leprosy colony in Maharashtra, India in 2010.

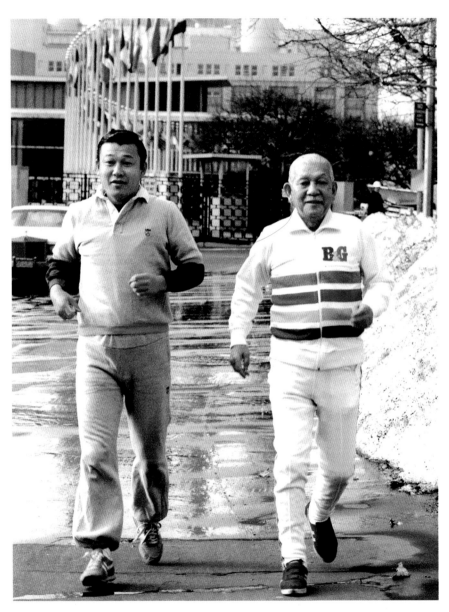

7. Ryoichi and Yohei Sasakawa jogging in front of the headquarters of the United Nations, New York (1980s).

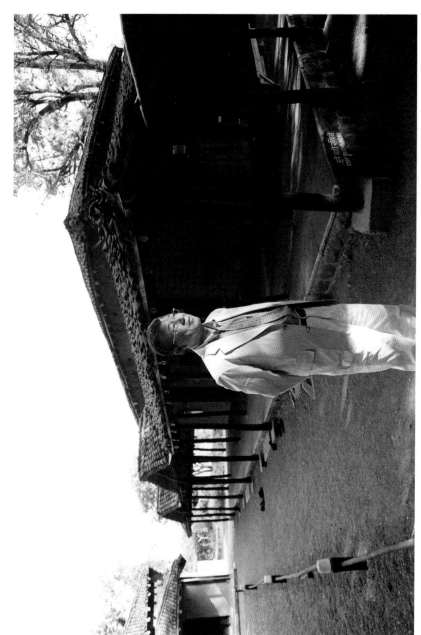

8. Yohei Sasakawa at Gandhi Sevagram Ashram, Maharashtra, India, in 2003.

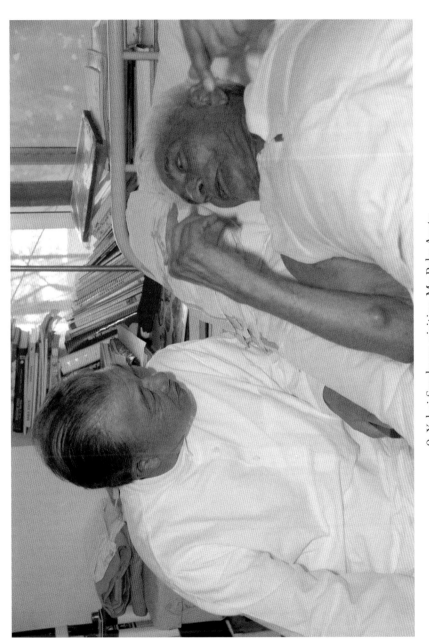

9. Yohei Sasakawa visiting Mr Baba Amte.

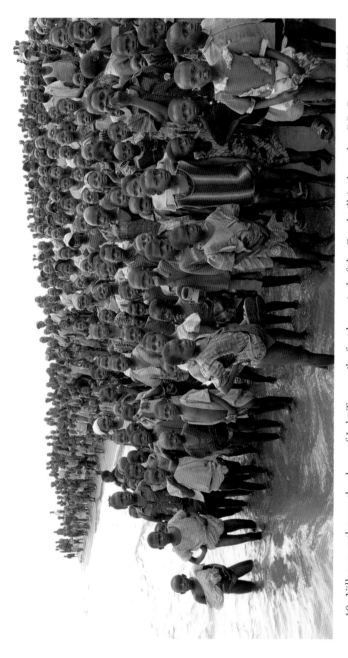

10. Villagers gather on the shore of Lake Tanganyika for the arrival of the Goodwill Ambassador, DR Congo, 2008.

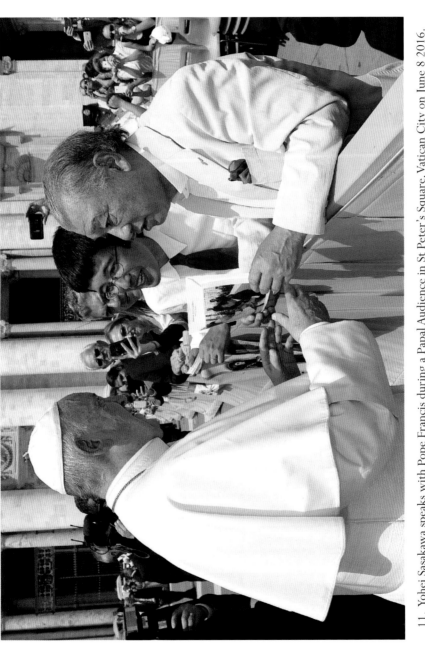

11. Yohei Sasakawa speaks with Pope Francis during a Papal Audience in St Peter's Square, Vatican City on June 8 2016.

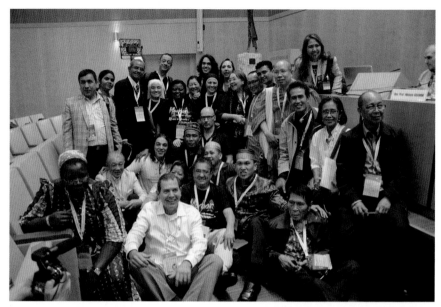

12. People of different cultures and faiths come together at the Vatican for the symposium 'Towards Holistic Care for People with Hansen's Disease, Respecting their Dignity' in 2016.

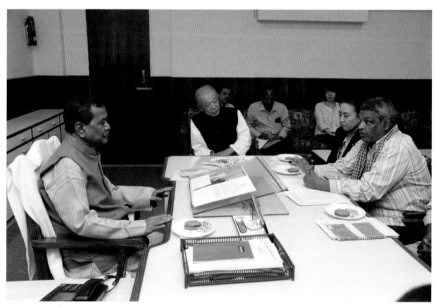

13. APAL's State leader for Odisha, Mr Umesh Nayak presents Odisha's Health Minister Dr Pradip Kumar Amat with a petition.

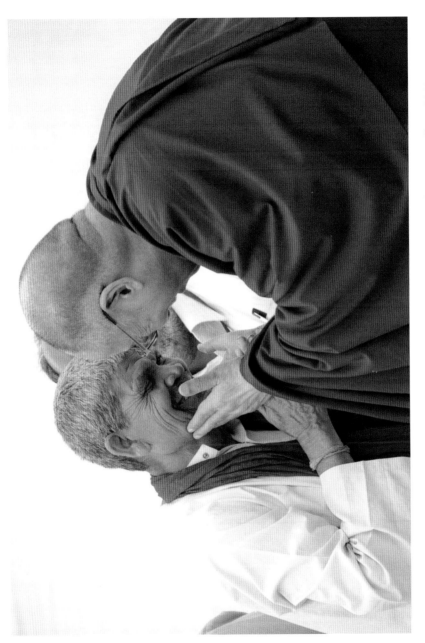

14. His Holiness the 14th Dalai Lama visiting the Tahirpur Leprosy Complex, New Delhi in 2014.

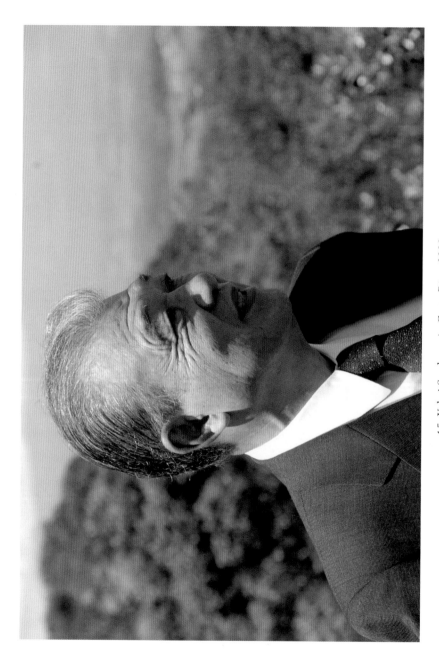

15. Yohei Sasakawa in Costa Rica, 2008.

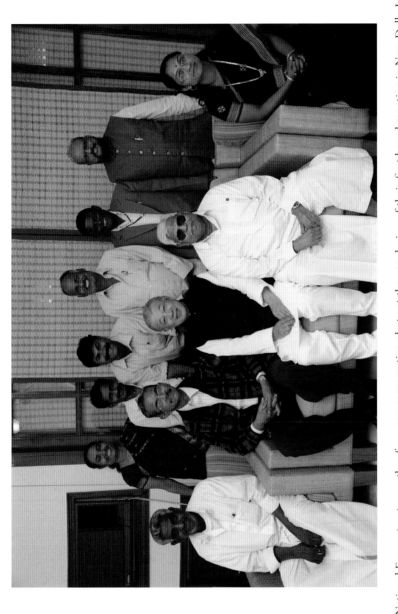

16. The National Forum trustees gather for a commemorative photo at the conclusion of their first board meeting in New Delhi, India. Back row (left to right): Lourdes Nevis Mary, Sarang Sudam Gaidhane, Rambarai Sah, Vagavathali Narasappa, G. Venugopal, Uday Thakar; Front row: A. Prakkasam, Dr. P.K. Gopal (chairman), Yohei Sasakawa, Bhimrao Madhale, Maya Ranavare, 2011.

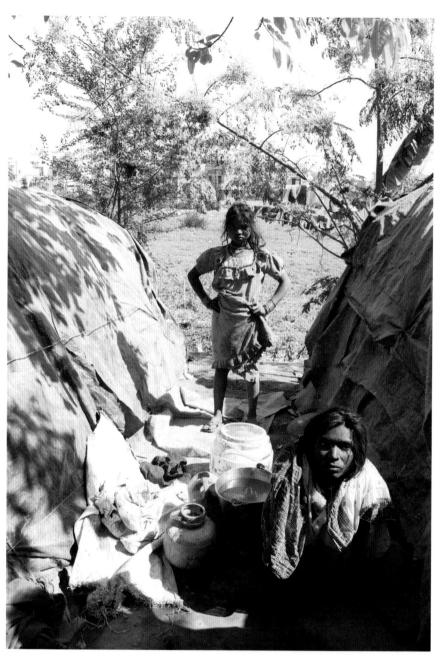

17. In Jitwarpur leprosy colony in Samstipur, Bihar State, India. Living also with persons with disabilities and other of society's poorer members, their conditions were very basic and it brought home to me the extent of the challenges that remain to improve the lives of persons in these colonies, 2011.

should take, and among the issues raised were investigating the conditions at leprosy colonies around the nation, creating a database, setting up a website, forming a strategy for fundraising, and establishing an advisory committee. Regarding fundraising, personally I sought to raise locally an amount equal to the US$10 million being contributed by the Nippon Foundation.

According to Mr. Das, who, as Director-General of CII, had long pushed for social contributions by his country's corporate sector, India's business community, as part of its commitments to social improvement, was already extending small loans to unskilled labourers who wished to undergo vocational training or to people who aspired to start their own companies. Mr. Das added that Indian businesses also frequently dispatched advisors to offer advice free of charge. In his view, given the existence of organizations already possessing expertise and a solid track record in these areas, S-ILF would do best by serving as an intermediary—a catalyst—linking organizations possessing information, technology and resources with the nation's leprosy colonies.

The trend toward corporate social responsibility actions of these kinds in India owes much to the country's economic strides of recent years. Compared to the corporate philanthropy that proliferated in Japan during the era of the "bubble" economy, which focused on supporting cultural and artistic pursuits, the activities being undertaken by India's business community struck me as far more practical and sensible. I couldn't but feel that India is well ahead of Japan as a civil society.

In October 2007 we organized meetings in Delhi and Mumbai targeted at spreading an understanding of S-ILF's founding objectives among India's business community, the media, people in government and so on, and to request their cooperation in the future.

The ceremony in Delhi was attended by Dr. A.P.J. Abdul Kalam, who had served as India's President until as recently as that July. Dr. Kalam told the assembled audience that the existence of leprosy colonies was unpardonable, and he expressed the hope that, with time, colonies would one day cease to exist. That evening a gathering was held for India's political and business leaders. Among the attendees was the Union Minister of Finance, P. Chidambaram, who pledged his support for S-ILF's undertakings.

Attending the ceremony in Mumbai was Jamshyd Godrej, former chairman of the Godrej Group, one of India's most prominent industrial conglomerates, who addressed the audience as representative of the country's business community. Given Mumbai's position as the headquarters for many of India's major corporate head offices, many members of the business community were present.

NO MATTER WHERE THE JOURNEY TAKES ME

Receipt of International Gandhi Award, making acquaintance of Baba Amte

In July 2007 I was blessed with the honour of receiving the International Gandhi Award, an accolade bestowed in recognition of my many years of contribution to leprosy work. I was the first Japanese to receive this coveted award, one of the most prestigious of its kind in the world.

The award ceremony took place in the city of Wardha in Maharashtra state. This was the location of the first All-India Leprosy Workers' Conference. Held in 1947, it brought together those engaged in leprosy work as well as others involved in Gandhi's Constructive Programme.

In my acceptance speech, I spoke of the need to "change society, where a discriminatory attitude pervades", making reference to Gandhi's famous words that "a disease of the mind is far more dangerous than physical disease", for I regard social discrimination as a disease.

During my stay in Wardha, where in July the temperature was hovering above 40 degrees, I was eager to pay a second visit to Gandhi's ashram. I found that nothing had changed since my previous visit in December 2003: the ashram was still a haven of tranquil serenity. I paused for some time in the shade created by the huge sal tree looming above me.

More than half a century had passed since Gandhi expressed his deep anguish over the leprosy problem. Yet in spite of the tremendous efforts and contributions made by so many people in the interim, I mulled over how this disease was still causing unspeakable suffering for those it affected and their family members because of the stigma attached to it. A disease of the mind is not easily cured. I pondered how I, like Gandhi, must maintain, with patience and a quiet heart, my unrelenting resolve to improve the situation for people affected by leprosy.

Standing on the ground where Gandhi had stood, I felt as if I could hear his voice, that of the "father of India", speaking to me.

In initiating S-ILF's activities on a full scale, I took numerous hints from the work being performed at Anandwan, a community rehabilitation centre for people affected by leprosy and the disabled. After the award ceremony in Wardha, I proceeded to fulfil a long-embraced desire to visit Anandwan, where I had the good fortune to meet Baba Amte, the social activist who had brilliantly demonstrated that it is possible to create an economically indepen-dent community free of prejudice and discrimination.

I first learned of Baba Amte's work from the Dalai Lama. His Holiness had told me that if I intended to carry out my activities in India, I should try by all means to meet Baba Amte. He added that he had visited Baba Amte and stayed with more than once.

INDIA, LAND OF "MOTHER GANGES"

When I met him in 2007, Baba Amte was 93 and nearly bedridden. All the same, I found him looking quite robust, and he said that in spite of having spent many years lying on his bed, his legs still retained their strength. He stretched out his hand—a very large hand, I discovered—to welcome me. To get around the facility where he was being cared for, he used a specially equipped bed-on-wheels; his spine had been injured from heavy labour he had performed as a young man. As he used no dentures, his speech was at times difficult for me to comprehend, but his son, Dr. Vikas Amte, kindly helped to "interpret". Baba Amte, who was also a philosopher, offered me a great number of words of inspiration and encouragement.

Baba Amte was born in 1914 into a family of considerable wealth. After receiving an education of the kind only available to India's elite, he became a lawyer. Then one day he had an experience that was to change his life. He passed a leprosy patient in the street who was on the verge of dying, and Amte found the sight so frightening that he panicked and quickly fled the scene.

After he regained his composure, he began questioning what he had done. "If I had a leprosy patient in my family, would I have fled like that, doing nothing to help?" Feeling shame at how he had behaved, he decided to become involved in activities to support the cause of leprosy. This commitment ultimately led to his creation, in Warora (Maharashtra), of a community where leprosy patients could live at peace. He named the community Anandwan, meaning "Forest of Joy".

In India's caste system, there exist numerous sub-castes—said to number anywhere between 3,000 and 3,500—consisting of groups of individuals who by heredity engage in a particular occupation. Among the many sub-castes, the lowest of the low is populated by those who work in collecting night soil. Even today, there are many individuals, especially in rural areas, who make their livelihood, as did their forefathers, by collecting human waste.

Baba Amte once formed a union of those who belonged to this sub-caste at the nadir of Indian society, in recognition of which his country's President referred to him as the "king of scavengers". Needless to say, Baba Amte was not one to be perturbed by being called such a nickname.

Baba Amte, along with his family members spanning three generations, lived at Anandwan in the company of some five thousand of India's less fortunate. Besides leprosy patients, the community welcomed people with physical disabilities. They all shared the sorrowful experience of having been abandoned by their families, and came to Anandwan seeking a ray of hope, no matter how dim.

Anandwan is large—some 176 hectares in all—and its residents eke out their livelihoods by farming the land or working in any of the various factories

121

on the premises: a sewing factory, printing factory, carpet factory, brick factory, crafts centre, metalworks, and factories making plastics or recycling tyres. The community is also home to a bank, post office, shops, and a hospital and university both operated by the community itself. In this way, Anandwan is a full-fledged, self-contained town in its own right.

I decided to pay a visit to the community barbershop, operated by a man affected by leprosy, to have a shave. The barber was altogether unruffled by the appearance of this unusual customer, and after adjusting my head to make sure my neck was at just the right angle, he rubbed soap on my face with his calloused hands and immediately got to work. He proceeded to shave me with a dull blade, massaged my scalp until it hurt, and finally wiped my face with a cloth that was hardly what one would call clean. I bore it all without saying a word. Watching the whole procedure, Dr. Vikas clapped his hand with joy. "Now that was brave of you!" he said with glee.

I asked Baba's wife what it had been like at Anandwan when it was first started. She described how Baba and the family had settled in what was then an untamed forest, together with six leprosy patients and one cow. The area was rife with leopards, poisonous snakes, scorpions and other nasty creatures, and Mrs. Amte related how she had personally witnessed four dogs being attacked by a leopard. Life in those days was frightening to the core, she said; but the calm way she spoke gave no trace of her having experienced such harsh times. She exuded an air of tranquil dignity and robust spirit.

"As a young man Baba wore his hair very long, like an ascetic. He wasn't attractive at all, and everyone was opposed to my marrying him!"

"So he owes his worldwide respect entirely to his wife, right?"

"To be sure!"

With that, Mrs. Amte laughed loudly with great joy.

"Mr. Sasakawa, please go to my husband's bedside and tell him what you just told me!"

This time she smiled a broad smile.

For more than half a century since its foundation, Anandwan has continuously functioned as a "shelter" protecting India's most vulnerable citizens who, even today, face intense public prejudice and discrimination. The significance of the community's existence truly defies description. Seeing it with my own eyes, I was both astonished and impressed at the work that had been achieved by Baba Amte and his family in creating a totally self-reliant and self-sufficient system on a modest scale.

"Our mission is to close Anandwan," Dr. Vikas noted. "In other words, to create a society in which Anandwan will no longer be necessary." Despite having long carried out activities to eliminate leprosy by using different methods, I was in full agreement with those sentiments. The ultimate goal of our activities isn't to protect people affected by leprosy from prejudice and discrimination, but rather to see a world in which such prejudice and discrimination will have vanished.

To borrow Vikas's words, our mission is to close the Sasakawa-India Leprosy Foundation: in other words, to create a society in which S-ILF will no longer be needed.

Embraced by the Flow of the Ganges

Ripple effect: the subsequent years of the National Forum and S-ILF

When a pebble is dropped into a calm pool of water, small ripples appear that gradually spread in concentric circles.

Throughout my life, through a variety of support activities I have witnessed how many different people—not only those in any way affected by leprosy—go about living their lives. To lend support to someone or to something is, to my mind, like tossing a small pebble into a pool of water. Dropping sand into water is too "weak" to cause ripples. Hurling a big rock will see it merely sink to the bottom, again giving rise to no ripples. Putting one's hand in the water is of no effect, and diving into the water oneself isn't feasible.

To generate ripples, it's necessary to toss in a pebble of just the right size with just the right timing. Then once you confirm that beautiful ripples have been set in motion, you then set out looking for another place to toss another pebble.

I have supported efforts to eliminate leprosy in India, increasingly addressed the human rights issues of people affected by leprosy and their family members, and formed networks that connect them. In retrospect, until around 2008 what I did was indeed to toss small pebbles into water at various locations. And thanks to the efforts made by the people I worked with and those who cooperated in my mission, beautiful ripples were set in motion at each place where our pebbles were tossed.

Beginning in 2009, those ripples then began spreading, as I will now describe.

In late February and early March 2009 I visited Lucknow, the capital of Uttar Pradesh state. Uttar Pradesh is India's largest state, with a population estimated at 180 million. Lucknow is a city rich in history, with many notable sites that date back to the time when the area was ruled by Nawabs, Muslim royalty, in the eighteenth to nineteenth centuries. My visit was occasioned by the holding of the National Forum Northern Regional Conference, the first such gathering in India's north.

The National Forum had seen steady growth since its first convention back in 2005. The forums were widely attended by people affected by leprosy and they served as venues where participants exchanged information and deepened their ties. In the process, the scope of their activities, targeting social and economic improvements, had steadily expanded.

In all, the Northern Regional Conference brought together approximately 330 representatives of northern India's leprosy colonies spread across ten states including not only Uttar Pradesh but also Delhi, Madhya Pradesh and Bihar. In contrast to previous forums that were attended almost exclusively by men of senior age, at the gathering at Lucknow females and young participants made up roughly 30% of the participants. This was a most welcome change.

The conference was opened by the Health Minister of Uttar Pradesh, Anant Kumar Mishra. Listening to his remarks, and watching how various people affected by leprosy took to the podium and made their presentations, I felt deeply that, thanks to the superb meshing of the efforts made by people affected by leprosy, the backing provided by enlightened political leaders and the support extended by NGOs, the environment surrounding India's leprosy colonies showed signs of moving in the right direction.

Ahead of the conference, S-ILF had approved its first ten grants for microfinancing, and the award certificates had been bestowed on the chosen recipients. The grants were awarded to residents of colonies for a variety of projects—including dairy farming, candle-making and retailing—in the states of Madhya Pradesh, Uttarakhand and Tamil Nadu. The grants were in amounts ranging from 23,500 to 309,000 rupees (approx. US$375 to $5,000)—considerable sums in a country where so many millions live on the equivalent of less than US$1 a day.

Together with the National Forum, steady strides were also being made in advancing the work performed by S-ILF.

In late January 2010, the first Southern Regional Conference of the National Forum was held at a hotel in the city of Chennai. The conference was attended by some 350 representatives of colonies in India's southern states of Tamil Nadu, Kerala, Karnataka and Andhra Pradesh.

The conference focused on the question of how to improve the social and economic positions of people affected by leprosy, and participants from various social positions exchanged a wealth of information. Geetha Jeevan, the Minister for Social Welfare in Tamil Nadu state, told the audience that leprosy was like any other disease in that it could be contracted by anyone, and she pledged that her state government would continue to provide support for the rehabilitation of people affected by leprosy as well as to the disabled, all people in vulnerable positions, and females in need. Those affected by leprosy in the audience were greatly encouraged by her words, and they roundly applauded her with renewed hope for their states and the national government to follow through with the actions of Ms. Jeevan.

By this point in time the National Forum had begun to demonstrate power to move India's political leaders and administrative bodies. Indeed, the Forum's growth was truly remarkable. Among the various speeches offered by colony representatives that day, one made a profound impression on me in particular. "In the old days we had no medicine for leprosy and suffered," the speaker said. "Even now we have many problems, but seeing the happy faces of all of you who have gathered here today makes me happier than anything. There are things that we, ourselves, should be able to accomplish."

These words bespeak the fact that people affected by leprosy, the very people who are being supported, are themselves beginning to undergo changes. Changes in the people directly affected by leprosy will surely constitute a major force in fundamentally resolving the many issues created by this disease.

Following the conference in Chennai, I paid a visit to the Balaramapuram colony in the Villivakkam area of the city. The colony had been founded around 1980 and its living conditions were gradually being improved with support from NGOs and the government. This was my third time visiting it, and each time I noticed new buildings and saw improvements in the lives of the colony's residents. The colony is home to some one hundred households, approximately 300 people in all, with healthy residents and people affected by leprosy living all together. In this way, by the time of my visit in early 2010 Balaramapuram / Villivakkam had grown into an integrated community.

The leader of the Villivakkam colony was Mr. A. Prakasam, who himself was affected by leprosy. Mr. Prakasam had at one time suffered great hardship begging for his living, but now he was living happily together with his children and grandchildren. A man with strong leadership qualities, he had united all the colonies in Tamil Nadu state and served for two decades as president of the Tamil Nadu Leprosy Patients' Rehabilitation Guild, devoting himself indefatigably to restoring the dignity of people affected by leprosy.

At Balaramapuram we conducted a study of the people who had received microloans from S-ILF. Under the guidance of experts, the recipients had drawn up business plans based on which the colony was now producing and selling items including clothing, plastic products and auto parts. With great pride they showed me their wares—clothes, toys, cooking pots, shoes—all of good quality. A pair of sandals was being sold for 100 rupees (approx. US$1.60) and a plastic cooking pot for 400 rupees.

I asked one man who operated a retail shop in the colony how he was getting along. He said that after expenses his shop generated a monthly profit of around 3,000 rupees (US$50), which, he noted with pleasure, was sufficient to enable him to send his two children to school. I also spoke with a woman who was selling saris, scarves and the like. She explained how she always works very hard to create products that will give pleasure to her customers, doing so by continually looking into what is currently in fashion and which things are selling best. I said it must be difficult making a good profit since her customers must always be trying to reduce the price. "Not so," she replied with robust confidence. "Normally I deal in cash, and to prevent my customers from trying to cut the price I allow them to pay in two instalments."

Seeing the professional way in which the recipients of SILF's microloans were going about their businesses, I felt that the work being done by SILF was clearly producing positive results.

I next paid a visit to the Balpart colony, about 30 minutes away by car. This is a colony of about 35 households, some 110 residents in all, which developed with support from a Christian charity. The homes in that colony were built by young people who learned how to build with support from the charity. The colony's financial situation was quite severe, however, and every day nearly one in every ten residents left the grounds and went by train to one of Chennai's temples to beg—an effort that brought in approximately 50 rupees, i.e. less than the equivalent of US$1. Some families raised goats and sold their milk, but even they lived a hand-to-mouth existence.

These challenges aside, people came and asked about applying for microfinancing from S-ILF, determined to start a business raising livestock. Here too, I could sense that the small pebble I had tossed into the waters was beginning, ever so quietly, to set ripples in motion.

While in Chennai, I was also able to take part in a cultural event organized by the National Forum that occurs each year on the last Sunday in January, in tandem with World Leprosy Day. The proceedings took place in an open air theatre that had been constructed in Gandhi's memory, and on stage the children and grandchildren of people affected by leprosy living in Chennai's various colonies sang and danced with great enjoyment. Young people also performed a magic show, while other participants introduced the diversity of India's languages and cultures, all to the accompaniment of music, making for a very lively display.

One young girl whose grandfather was affected by leprosy spoke with passion about her dream for the future. "I want to become a doctor," she related, "so I can help people who suffer from sicknesses the way my grand-father once did."

Children are the hopes and dreams of the future. Wherever I go, whenever I have the opportunity, I always ask them what they want to become in the future. Many reply that they would like to be a doctor or a nurse or a teacher. These are the ardent dreams of children who have grown up watching their parents struggling.

Initiatives in India's poorest state: Bihar, April 2010

Even since India attained the elimination target at the national level, there are still regions of the country where the prevalence rate of leprosy remains high. Visiting such areas and taking initiatives to advance moves toward eliminating the disease in those regions is a vital part of my mission as Goodwill Ambassador for Leprosy Elimination.

A state that has long weighed heavily on my mind is Bihar, where reaching and sustaining the elimination of leprosy has remained an elusive goal. Bihar is located in north-east India along the border with Nepal. In ancient times, when it was known as Magadha, it prospered as the Maurya empire. Today Bihar is one of India's, and the world's, foremost pilgrimage destinations, for the state is home to Bodhgaya, where Prince Siddhartha Gautama attained enlightenment and became the Buddha.

Its historical legacy and current fame aside—and with a population as large as Japan—Bihar detected over 21,000 new cases of leprosy in 2016–2017, the most of any state. Given the characteristically poor living standards in the region, people affected by leprosy suffer severe discrimination and are forced to live on the fringes of society, or worse.

In April 2010 I visited Bihar to undertake an investigation of the situation of the state's leprosy colonies. Leaving the sweltering heat of Delhi behind me, I took a night flight to Patna, the state capital. Upon disembarking I encountered heat even more oppressive than in Delhi. In the daytime, the temperature reached 45 degrees and the sun beat down mercilessly, falling on one's skin with stinging intensity. With the cooperation of Bihar Kustha Kalyan Mahasangh (BKKM), an umbrella group of associations of people affected by leprosy in the state, I visited three colonies in the East Champaran district, some two hours by car from Patna.

The first colony, at Motipur, was home to 55 households with a total population of 158, including 40 people affected by leprosy. On arrival I noticed the voices of children not far away, and on going to see what they were doing I discovered a group of youngsters all neatly lined up in the corridor of a school building half exposed to the elements, reading aloud from their textbooks. With help from an NGO, a classroom had been built inside the colony, a response to the discrimination such students would otherwise face if they attended the local public school. The residents of the colony were living in simple straw huts—huts that inevitably leaked in the rain as they deteriorated over time.

According to the colony's leader, the colony was receiving a modicum of assistance from the government, but the number of families issued with certificates giving low-income families free access to essential goods was limited. Particularly egregious was the circumstance that people affected by leprosy were, in spite of their disabilities, barred from receiving the special allowances that are normally granted to the disabled. I was also told that special allowances paid to the elderly were habitually in arrears.

Under these circumstances, the majority of Motipur's residents were compelled to resort to begging. Needless to say, I found no one who was hopeful of getting a job and becoming self-reliant.

I next visited the colony at Chakia, where the inhabitants also got along by begging. Chakia was a small colony: just 45 residents in 35 households. The colony had been devastated by flooding on numerous occasions, especially in the great flood that swept through in 2009, in which nearly all the houses were washed away. In the aftermath, the Sasakawa Memorial Health Foundation had provided support for the colony's recovery. But the temporary "homes" that were built at the time by the roadside even lacked toilets; and at the time of my visit in April 2010, although there were plans to build toilets within the colony, I was told that they were stalled because of opposition from nearby businesses. And to compound matters, the colony's residents were now being pressed to relocate because of plans to widen the road, and they were in the midst of pressing the government to ensure that as a substitute they would receive another plot of land close by. In the face of this threat to their very lives, the residents of Chakia affected by leprosy all showed visible anxiety, casting a dark pall of depression over the entire colony.

The third of the three colonies I visited was in Pipra, a small community of 13 households of 22 inhabitants. Earlier that year Pipra had been the scene of a tragedy of symbolic significance: the death of a young boy, just 5 years old, in an arson attack on the colony perpetrated by a local landowner who was seeking to evict residents from the property, causing the destruction of several homes. Through the newly established BKKM, working in cooperation with Bihar state representatives and leaders from the National Forum, negotiations were conducted with police and government officers, resulting in the payment of 100,000 rupees (approx. US$1,600) in compensation and a promise to be given nearby land on which the government pledged to construct new housing for the colony's inhabitants. There was no guarantee, however, that such promises would actually be carried out, especially given the large number of instances in India where pledges of this sort ultimately prove empty.

Astonishingly, in spite of the pathetic state of Bihar's leprosy colonies as demonstrated by what I personally witnessed in Motipur, Chakia and Pipra, at the time of my visit the governmental post that oversees issues relating to leprosy in the state was vacant. Together with representatives from BKKM, I went to visit the State Minister of Health, to urge that an outstanding person fill the position of state leprosy officer and to ask for support to improve the living conditions in the state's colonies. I not only received a positive response from the Health Minister; I also came away with a promise from the top administrator in the ministry concerning the issue of special allowances for people affected by leprosy and the housing issue. He gave me his word that if detailed materials and a list of people hoping to receive special allowances were brought to him within two weeks, he would attend to those matters without delay.

I immediately discussed what had transpired with the relevant persons and asked them to draw up a list of people affected by leprosy who were living in Bihar together with a report on the living conditions in each of the state's colonies. To cover the costs involved, I provided US$1,000 from my personal funds. I promised to return to India when the requisite materials were ready for submission and to accompany them when they submitted them to the Health Minister, and returned to Japan for the time being.

Over the next two weeks seven representatives of BKKM spread out over the entire length and breadth of Bihar, a state with a land area larger than Portugal or Hungary, and gathered the information required of them, often forgoing sleep in order to complete their task to their full satisfaction. Upon receiving word that their investigations had been completed, I immediately returned to Bihar.

I was astonished at the depth and detail of their findings. The report covered a total of 997 households living in 63 colonies, and it recorded details concerning lands and housing, family composition, and whether a family was receiving a special allowance or not. In the space of less than a month the team members had personally visited each and every home. When I joined up with them, they were brimming with self-confidence. "I haven't had time to see my wife in weeks!" one of them joked.

With the thick report of the team's findings in hand, together we went to meet state officials for a second time. This time we were granted meetings with a number of people in high positions, including Deputy Chief Minister Sushil Kumar Modi, whom I had been unable to meet on my previous visit. When I went to meet Mr. Modi, I took along a number of people affected by leprosy. They were the principals in this drama and I wanted them to do the talking. My decision to take them along and have them speak was a spontaneous one—we had not discussed the matter in advance; and they were wholly taken by surprise, flabbergasted to the point of being unable to speak properly in the presence of the distinguished Deputy Chief Minister.

Mr. Modi, however, appeared to be deeply moved as he pored over the report these people affected by leprosy had prepared. He stated that the government of Bihar had actually conducted studies concerning leprosy in the state in the past, but he voiced astonishment at the report he had just been given, which far exceeded those earlier official studies both in volume and quality. He also stated that there was great significance in the fact that the report had been researched and compiled by people affected by leprosy themselves.

The efforts they had made quickly bore fruit. Mr. Modi replied on the spot that the land and special allowance issues would be resolvable within one month's time.

This was actually not the first time I had met Mr. Modi, although the previous occasion had been back in 2003, seven years earlier. The passage of time notwithstanding, Mr. Modi remembered in remarkable detail how my father, Ryoichi Sasakawa, had come to address the issues concerning leprosy in the first place.

The outcome of our visit, and the fact that the people, on their own, had succeeded in winning a pledge of support and cooperation from a high official in their state government, served as great encouragement to the leaders of people affected by leprosy in Bihar. What's more, in the course of conducting their investigations using their own feet, hands, eyes and ears, a sense of solidarity had developed among them, together with an almost palpable sense of responsibility as leaders. I felt that if this could happen in Bihar, one of India's poorest states, then it should be possible in other states too. As I recount later, this proved to be the case.

Addressing further issues, February 2011

On 21 February 2011 the National Forum underwent a change in status to an incorporated body. In accordance with its articles of incorporation, the first board meeting was held on 26 February in Delhi. Dr. P.K. Gopal was selected to fill the position of chairman, while I accepted an appointment as advisor.

At the board meeting a motion was passed defining three overriding objectives of the National Forum's activities: to strengthen the organization at the local level, to cultivate young leaders, and to create a special allowance system for persons affected by leprosy. None of these tasks would be easy to achieve, but they all demanded to be addressed with great urgency.

Strengthening the organization at the local level referred specifically to forming the underlying structure for the National Forum's activities at the state level, in the context of India's sustained moves toward decentralization of power.

Cultivating young leaders was a prime necessity in order that the issues surrounding leprosy, defying quick resolution, might be addressed by succeeding generations. All the core members of the National Forum were advancing in years, as indeed I was. Given that cultivating able human resources takes time, there was no time to be lost in this respect.

Creating a special allowance system for people affected by leprosy was necessitated by the circumstances concerning special allowances in India at the time. Although national and state special allowance systems were in place for the disabled and the elderly, a corresponding system for people affected by leprosy existed only in a limited number of locations: for example, in Delhi and Uttarakhand state. In October 2008 the Rajya Sabha Committee on Petitions had tabled a report calling for the establishment in all states of a special allowance for people affected by leprosy with a disbursement amount of 2,000 rupees per month (approx. US$32). I was determined to see that such a scheme was carried out and further expanded.

In order to address these various issues, immediately after the board meeting concluded I set about launching a non-partisan group of India's parliamentarians to back the social rehabilitation of the country's people affected by leprosy.

Losing no time, I flew immediately from Delhi to Patna, capital of Bihar, in the east. As described above, the previous year I had met with the state's Deputy Chief Minister, Sushil Kumar Modi, and received a favourable response from him. After my visit Mr. Modi had become involved in general elections and other duties, and unfortunately no progress in improving the treatment of people affected by leprosy had been made of the kind we had hoped for. I decided to go to Patna again, to try to get things moving again.

In Patna I was granted opportunities to meet with Sanjay Kumar, executive director for Bihar of the National Rural Health Mission, Ganga Prasad, Deputy Speaker of the Bihar Legislative Council, and once again Deputy

Chief Minister Sushil Kumar Modi. During our meeting Mr. Modi immediately got on the phone and called the person in charge at the Ministry of Social Welfare and instructed him to put together a concrete special allowance plan. He also promised me he would speak with the Chief Minister about the matter. These were the greatest results to emerge from this visit to Bihar.

Mr. Modi also made arrangements for me to meet with Bihar's Minister of Health, Ashwini Kumar Choubey. We presented him with a list of specific requests: the issuing to people affected by leprosy of official certificates enabling them to receive a special allowance, twice-weekly visits by medical staff to the state's colonies, distribution of protective footwear to the disabled, and disbursement of medical benefits. Mr. Choubey's response was encouraging.

In my experience I have found that Indian officials give serious consideration to the matters set before them by visitors from abroad, and thus I feel this is the greatest function I can fulfil, by going to India to discuss issues in person.

I next called on the Bihar branch of the UK-based Leprosy Relief Association (LEPRA), where I received a detailed briefing on leprosy in the state. I was told that for every 10,000 people in Bihar there are 1.08 registered patients, with the number of new patients topping 20,000 a year, of which some 16% are children. The ratio of new registrants who show symptoms of disability is quite low, however, less than 2%, a relatively positive statistic attributable to the disease's early detection.

While in Bihar I was escorted to see Tajpur Hospital, a facility whose leprosy ward is operated by LEPRA. Tajpur Hospital is a publicly funded institution located some two and a half hours by car north-east of Patna. At the time of my visit, its coverage area encompassed 150 villages with a total population of 150,000. Every month the hospital took in an average of between four and five new patients. Early detection of the disease and prevention of disability development were supported by a team of approximately 150 volunteers who made regular rounds of the villages. The hospital also operated a programme under which 20 to 30 persons affected by leprosy came twice each month for treatment of foot ulcerations.

There are still colonies in a dire situation, however, as illustrated by the Jitwarpur colony in the city of Samastipur, which is another half-hour by car beyond the Tajpur Hospital. The colony consisted of eight families of people affected by leprosy and sixteen families with disabilities all packed densely into a narrow strip of land alongside a road. They had been relocated to this location around 2001 from their former site, which had been next to railway tracks by a train station. In contrast to many of India's colonies of people affected by leprosy whose living environment had gradually improved thanks to various support programmes, the "houses" in the Jitwarpur colony were crude at best, mere tents forever beset by dust from the road. It was easy to assume that the people here eked out their living from begging, but I was too appalled—and deeply saddened—by the sight of their situation to ask them for confirmation of my suspicions.

After the National Forum had become an incorporated body, I had a sense that our activities in India had finally made significant progress; but from this trip to Bihar and what I witnessed there, it struck me deeply that the severe realities of India still waited to be addressed, just as at the outset.

In 2013, the special allowance issue in Bihar was finally resolved. It took three years' time from submission of the petition on this matter, but a major success had been achieved and the monthly special allowance was increased from 200 rupees to 1,800 rupees. This success scored in Bihar was to give great impetus to corresponding moves under way in other states.

Going forward, the goal will be to give hope to people affected by leprosy who currently have no alternative but to beg for their subsistence, and open up paths that will lead them to self-reliance.

Subsequent development of the National Forum as the Association of People Affected by Leprosy

Having assumed the role early in 2011, Dr. P.K. Gopal resigned his position as chairman of the National Forum later the same year and became the organization's advisor, whereupon the chairmanship was passed to Vagavathali Narsappa, an energetic man in his forties. Mr. Narsappa was born in a remote village in India's Karnataka state. At the age of 9, he began showing signs of leprosy, at which point the elders of his village declared he could no longer live among them. His family, having no recourse but to obey, tearfully removed the young Vagavathali from his home. It was at that moment, Mr. Narsappa says, that he became an outcast. His father took him to a hospital for leprosy patients in Andhra Pradesh state, and simply left him there.

"Even after I was treated, my family refused to take me back in," he relates. "I went on my own to a rehabilitation hospital, and there I was able to receive an education. When I went to take the entrance exam to a government school, I alone was prevented from entering the building and forced to take the exam outdoors, under a burning hot sun. Never in my entire life have I felt the bitter pain of discrimination as on that day. Today I'm able to live a happy life, with a wife and daughters, but I resolved to work for the salvation of other people affected by leprosy, and this has been the path my life has taken." Today, Mr. Narsappa is a leader in the movement to socially reintegrate and restore the dignity of people affected by leprosy. At the time he took up his post as chairman of the National Forum, he was unable to speak or read English fluently; but within several years, he became proficient, and today he is a core member of international conferences that bring together organizations of persons affected by leprosy from all over the world.

In 2011 the National Forum moved its office from Chennai to Hyderabad, where Mr. Narsappa resides, and changed its name to the Association of People Affected by Leprosy (APAL) in 2013.

In 2014, accompanied by Mr. Narsappa, I visited Uttar Pradesh, a state with a population of 210 million where, even now, more than 20,000 new cases of leprosy are discovered each year. After an initial meeting with the state's Principal Secretary (Health and Family Welfare), Arvind Kumar, I met with UP's Chief Minister, Akhilesh Yadav, together with Murari Sinha, secretary of a state-wide organization of persons affected by leprosy. Mr. Yadav had come to Japan more than ten years earlier under a programme of exchanges of Indian and Japanese parliamentarians conducted by the Sasakawa Peace Foundation, a sister organization of the Nippon Foundation, so we were old friends.

My meeting with Mr. Yadav took place with Principal Secretary Kumar present. I thanked the Chief Minister for the efforts he was making to address leprosy issues, and voiced a request that the state fill the post of leprosy officer in every district. I also brought up the example set by Bihar state concerning the special allowance granted to people affected by leprosy, and Mr. Narsappa and Mr. Kumar asked that the allowance in Uttar Pradesh be raised from its current level of 300 rupees. Mr. Yadav listened attentively to our appeals and agreed with everything we proposed. He demonstrated a strong commitment, adding that he would have the officials in charge take action, and he said he hoped we would monitor the situation going forward. I think his having visited Japan in the past was of benefit in this instance.

I next met with Uttar Pradesh Governor Ram Naik, who had previously served as India's Minister of Petroleum and Natural Gas. Here, I, along with a number of people affected by leprosy, made a similar request. The Governor is deeply committed to the well-being of people affected by leprosy and has played an active role in addressing the issues they face, as illustrated by his dedication to submitting a petition on steps needed for persons affected by leprosy to lead a dignified life to the Rajya Sabha Committee on Petitions in 2007, with the committee tabling its report in Parliament the following year. In retrospect, I had been deeply moved by the suggestion incorporated into that petition calling for the establishment in all states of a monthly special allowance of 2,000 rupees for persons affected by leprosy. I held high hopes that, with support from a man of Governor Naik's stature and influence, this would surely be realized.

After Uttar Pradesh, I proceeded to Delhi, where I was afforded an opportunity to meet with Prime Minister Narendra Modi. I had met with the Prime Minister just two months earlier during his visit to Tokyo. On that occasion, he had asked me why I had elected to work for the elimination of leprosy. I replied that I had taken over the unfulfilled dream my father had embraced: to eradicate leprosy and its attendant discrimination from the world. I told the Prime Minister of the leprosy hospital my father had founded in Agra. Prime Minister Modi had stated that he had deep respect for Mahatma Gandhi—noting that they shared roots in Gujarat state—and he spoke of his determination to devote himself to achieving Gandhi's dream of an India free of leprosy.

Only two months had passed since that meeting in Tokyo. On this occasion in Delhi, I was accompanied by Mr. Narsappa, representing APAL. 24 November 2014 will go down in history as the day the Prime Minister shook hands with this person affected by leprosy. I then made a request to Prime Minister Modi: to issue a message on World Leprosy Day in January stating that leprosy is a curable disease, that medicine is available free of charge, and that discrimination cannot be tolerated. Mr. Narsappa then sought the Prime Minister's support for improving the lives of people affected by leprosy.

Prime Minister Modi listened to us attentively. He then expressed appreciation for all I had done to eliminate leprosy in India, and he offered powerful words of assurance that he would carry forward measures against leprosy, especially in the states where it is endemic, and work to improve the lives of people affected by leprosy. After this meeting, under Prime Minister Modi's strong leadership, the activities of the Indian Government directed toward eliminating leprosy have made significant progress.

Returning to the matter of special allowances, based on the successes achieved in Bihar and Uttar Pradesh, after the 11th Global Appeal on 30 January, 2017, I travelled to Chhattisgarh, a state where leprosy remains endemic. Persons affected by leprosy there were demanding a monthly allowance of 5,000 rupees, and while I was somewhat taken aback by the scale of this demand, Ajay Chandrakar, Chhattisgarh's Minister of Health and Family Welfare, and Ramsheila Sahu, the State Minister of Women and Child Development and Social Welfare, promised the swift realization of this demand.

In March 2017 I visited another of India's endemic states, Odisha. Odisha is an impoverished state with a population of 44 million, close to that of Korea. On this occasion, together with the APAL state leader for Odisha, Umesh Nayak, I met with the Governor, Chief Minister, Health Minister, and representatives of several organizations dealing with issues affecting disabled persons. Our list of requests was wide-ranging, covering not only early detection of new cases but also addressing a plethora of issues impacting on leprosy colonies: land acquisition, access to electricity and water, dispatch of doctors to conduct medical examinations on a regular basis, provision of a special allowance as a way of preventing begging and the like.

Mr. Nayak earlier had lamented the treatment APAL had long received. "More than 20 times I've visited various offices to plead our case regarding these issues," he had told me, "but our petitions have always gone no further than the lowliest clerk." But this time he said he was so excited at the prospect of visiting the people in high office together with me that he had been unable to sleep the night before. Mr. Nayak, who represents 94 colonies within Odisha, feels all too keenly the heavy weight of his responsibility. During our meetings with officials, enormous beads of sweat flowed from his pores and his voice was faint, incongruous with the corpulent figure he presents.

After returning to Japan with a sense that my latest visit to India had been fruitful, I received happy word from Mr. Nayak. Something altogether unheard of had taken place: he had been invited to the Chief Minister's home and they had dined together. This bodes well for the future.

Progress of this kind notwithstanding, the mendicant ways of the people living in leprosy colonies in India die hard. To eliminate begging from India's colonies, I realize full well that yet more work remains to be done.

In Bihar it had taken three years to achieve, but the increase in the allowance paid to people affected by leprosy has made their lives easier. This is truly a source of immeasurable joy. In order to make things happen, it is necessary to negotiate tenaciously, repeatedly, and with patience. The main protagonists in these negotiations are people affected by leprosy. My role is to assist them from behind. This method had scored success in raising the special allowance in the states noted earlier. And in the process it has also instilled confidence and a sense of dignity in the persons affected by leprosy. People who have never been in a negotiating session before learn how to negotiate from scratch, to gather together the necessary information and materials, and to give precise explanations and precise answers to questions. It makes me happy to see the great progress they achieve with each new encounter. People affected by leprosy have begun standing on their own.

Mother Ganges, and all she means to me

By way of closing this introduction to my activities in India over the years, I would like to relate one day in particular which remains deeply etched in my memory.

INDIA, LAND OF "MOTHER GANGES"

In September 2008, after completing my work in Delhi I travelled to Varanasi, in Uttar Pradesh state. Varanasi, located alongside the Ganges, is a holy city for both Hindus and Buddhists.

As I was conducting elimination activities in India, I was eager to visit this city so closely entwined with the beliefs of the Indian people, especially their views toward life and death. For a long time I had dreamed of travelling down the Ganges by boat, and now finally I was given the opportunity to fulfil that wish.

I arrived very early in the morning, and already hordes of people were lining the river's banks. The riverbanks in Varanasi are home to close to a hundred "ghats", series of steps leading down to the river that serve as venues for prayer. Some of the ghats are also used by Hindus as cremation sites; the ashes of the deceased are dispersed into the Ganges, a process that Hindus believe will enable the departed to escape the cycle of rebirth. As a result people who are close to their end flock in great numbers to Varanasi from all over India. Those who are too poor to buy the firewood needed to build a pyre, young people who have died in an accident and children are set out to float, without cremation, in the waters of the Ganges.

Immediately to the side of these death rituals one finds people bathing or undergoing ablutions in the river. Not a few make a point of submerging to allow the "purifying" but turbid waters to cover their head and enter their mouth. By purifying their bodies in the Ganges, Hindus believe that any sins they have committed will be erased.

Domestic wastewater from Varanasi's residential quarters also flows directly into the Ganges. From a scientific viewpoint the river thus could not be more unsanitary; yet I was told that, strangely, almost no one who bathes in the Ganges becomes sick from the experience. Could the powers of this holy river truly be so great?

As I slowly sailed downstream in my small boat and watched the people bathing with such single-minded intent, I began to get the odd sensation that perhaps I had lost my way and entered the realm of the afterlife.

It was then that I noticed what appeared to be a large black shadow approaching me, floating on the water's surface. On close inspection I realized it was the carcass of a cow. Without thinking, I instinctively pulled back from the edge of the boat and turned my eyes away. The Ganges, however, just kept flowing on, as though nothing out of the ordinary had happened.

For thousands of years the Ganges has quietly accepted whatever has come its way: men and women, the young and the old, cows and dogs. Hundreds of millions if not billions of lives have been embraced by its waters. Now here

137

was I, similarly afloat in the great flow of the Ganges, and I felt a growing sense of peacefulness beyond explanation.

After this visit to Varanasi I continued to make frequent trips to India for conferences or workshops, for meetings with representatives of the media, or to travel to the country's leprosy colonies far and wide. And on many occasions I have found myself recalling the scenes I saw along the Ganges, in Varanasi, that unforgettable day in 2008.

Arising from the merging of waters tracing their origin to the faraway mountains of Nepal, the Ganges gathers momentum, swells to a river of grand proportions, and then continues its flow toward the sea, taking with it the souls of the multitudes.

Like the Ganges, the National Forum is also gathering momentum, I feel, and may one day change society. It may yet take another five or ten years, or maybe my entire lifetime, but I hope to watch over and support this organization's ongoing activities in every way and to the maximum extent I can.

I will continue my work, hand in hand with friends and colleagues, until the day that leprosy, together with the discrimination towards those who suffer from it, disappears from India completely.

Why? Because I am the son of Ryoichi Sasakawa. And because, in the same way that I love Japan, the country of my birth and upbringing, I deeply love India, a country that has placed challenges in front of me, but has also been a source of great joy and satisfaction as well. With the guidance of "Father" Gandhi and "Mother" Ganges, I will continue forward to complete the mission set out before me.

4

UNFORGETTABLE PLACES, UNFORGETTABLE FACES

Visits to Remote Islands

Keeping history alive

As the WHO Goodwill Ambassador for Leprosy Elimination, one of the principles I have always maintained when visiting leprosy-endemic countries is to meet with those in the highest positions of government and stress the importance of staying focused on leprosy and ensuring the human rights of people affected by the disease. At the same time, no matter how short my travel schedule and regardless of how difficult it might be to reach a location, I always make a point of taking as much time as possible to visit local hospitals and communities of people affected by leprosy to meet directly with patients and residents and offer words of encouragement.

Another matter I attach great importance to is to learn the history of leprosy in the country I am visiting, and call for the preservation of the sites and materials that would otherwise be doomed to disappear, pledging my support in that initiative. The way people affected by leprosy have been treated down the centuries represents a stain on humankind, and their history cannot be allowed to fade into oblivion if the mistakes of the past are not to be repeated.

Even among those who devote themselves to the cause of people affected by leprosy, there are some who believe that forgetting the past, letting the mistakes of history disappear, is necessary to order to build a new future. I believe they are wrong. I firmly believe rather that it is our inherent duty to elucidate the responsibilities and mission we are meant to fulfil today by squarely addressing the weighty history of discrimination committed since time began and confronting the discriminatory feelings that can take root in anyone at any time.

I came to firmly embrace this belief based on my numerous experiences seeing at first hand how leprosy historically equated with isolation, and isolation historically equated with sequestration on a remote island—a pattern that became evident in all corners of the world.

As I described in Chapter 1, until it became a curable disease, leprosy was greatly feared, leading those who contracted it to be ostracized and isolated. The many leprosariums that were created on remote islands are poignant symbols of the tragic history that has surrounded leprosy.

In this chapter my aim is to present a record of my visits to these islands of isolation and to describe what I experienced there.

Malta, an early example of leprosy vanquished

In late March 2004 I went to Malta to learn how it had succeeded in eradicating leprosy. I travelled in the company of Kazuko Yamaguchi, executive director of the Sasakawa Memorial Health Foundation and an expert on leprosy issues. A decade before multidrug therapy (MDT) was first recommended by the WHO as the appropriate treatment for leprosy, Malta began successfully treating leprosy patients with its own form of MDT. I had long been interested to learn more about how Malta went about this and the situation on the island since the last patient had been cured.

The Republic of Malta is an archipelago of several small islands located to the south of Italy, approximately 80 kilometres south of Sicily. Given its location virtually at the very center of the Mediterranean Sea, over the course of seven thousand years of history Malta has been visited by peoples of every description and has been a witness to the rise and fall of civilizations in Europe and all around the Mediterranean. In more recent times the country has achieved robust development both as a stopover point for ships and as a financial centre. It is also known as a holiday destination.

Malta is a fascinating country, home today to three World Heritage sites. It consists mainly of three islands: Malta, Gozo and Comino. Malta island in particular is blessed with a complexly formed shoreline along its southeastern coast that historically provided the ideal setting for a natural fortress. Here, traces remain of civilizations spanning the period from antiquity to the present.

A great stronghold was built on Malta by the Knights of the Order of St. John (later, the Knights of Malta), who were given the islands in 1530. From here they engaged in heroic battles to defend the island against invaders from the Ottoman Empire. In 1798 the Knights were forced to flee after losing to invading forces under Napoleon's command. Just two years later, however, this time the Napoleonic victors were sent packing by the British, and for the next 160 or so years Malta remained a British possession, a position that dragged the archipelago into two world wars. Finally, in 1964 Malta won its independence from the British. In 1974, as the Republic of Malta it became a member of the British Commonwealth.

When I visited this island nation with its complex and fascinating history for the first time in 2004, in addition to the capital city, Valletta, and the fortified Three Cities, my interest was especially piqued by Manoel Island, a small flat island situated in the bay south-east of Valletta. A quarantine centre was opened here in 1643. The island is located a mere 40 to 50 metres from the mainland and today it is connected to Valletta by a bridge, making it possible for the casual visitor to overlook the fact that Manoel is in fact an island. On the eastern side of Manoel rises a great fortress, below which, along the sea coast, is an unusual stone structure featuring a long arched colonnade. This is the quarantine centre, known as the Lazzaretto, built on the site more than 370 years ago.

Malta, given its strategically important location in the Mediterranean, has since antiquity been visited by passing ships that carried people, goods, animals and, not infrequently, pestilent diseases. Particularly in the Middle Ages, Europe was repeatedly racked by plague, and Malta, already the seat of the Knights of the Order of St. John, in response set up a quarantine station on an island away from the main island as a self-defensive measure. Called Lazzaretto, from the generic name given to such isolation facilities, the term can be traced linguistically to the parable of Lazarus the beggar in the Gospel of Luke.

Malta's medical history contains reports of leprosy patients throughout the seventeenth and eighteenth centuries. The number of patients is said to have increased in the second half of the nineteenth century, a trend largely attributed to the return of numerous Maltese from northern Africa coupled with the presence in Malta of some six thousand Indian soldiers sent by Britain at the time of the Russo-Turkish War of 1877–1878. This time frame coincides with the period when increasing numbers of leprosy patients were beginning to become a matter of concern at places all across the globe.

The British occupying Malta at the time believed that it was necessary, as in other territories in their empire, to isolate and confine the archipelago's leprosy patients. In 1893 an ordinance was promulgated to that effect and the British authorities set out to establish facilities appropriate for isolation. Initially, in 1899 a facility for men was created at the extant Asylum for the

Aged and Incurable—commonly known as the "Poor House"—located at Mgieret on the mainland. This was followed in 1912 by a facility there for women, firmly setting in place Malta's leprosy isolation policy. According to statistics for the year 1918, the number of leprosy patients then stood at 4.72 per 10,000 of the population.

Owing to the brevity of my visit, I was unable to trace the history of leprosy in Malta fully. Fortunately, however, I was given an opportunity to meet with Professor Victor Griffiths (1920–2014), Professor Emeritus at the University of Malta, who had previously been on the national committee in charge of forming policies to deal with leprosy. From his recollections and various materials he kindly showed me, I was able to glean a great deal about how Malta coped with leprosy in modern times.

According to Professor Griffiths, besides the pair of isolation centres on the main island already noted, an isolation facility had also been created on the island of Gozo, to the north, in 1937. The former centres later became St. Bartholomew Hospital while that on Gozo evolved into Sacred Heart Hospital. Malta's laws mandating compulsory isolation were in principle ended as early as 1953, however, following the development of drug treatments starting in the 1940s and in line with the general global trend. Subsequently leprosy came to be treated primarily on an outpatient basis, and all of Malta's leprosariums were closed by 1974. The earliest leprosarium previously located at the Poor House later became part of St. Vincent de Paul Residence, a care facility for the elderly inhabited by some one thousand residents at the time of my visit. The isolation wards that once existed have been removed without a trace.

Statistics for the year 1957, shortly after leprosy treatment shifted to an outpatient system, list the number of leprosy patients in Malta at 152, compared to a total population of 314,369. This is by no means a negligible quantity. The only drug treatment available at this time was dapsone, and treatment was said to be lengthy. Over time, though, cases of resistance to dapsone were reported, and specialists began investigations into a new method of chemotherapy. One such programme was the Malta Leprosy Eradication Project (MLEP).

MLEP was launched in 1972 under the leadership of Malta's health authority with support from the Sovereign Military Order of Malta, the German Leprosy Relief Association (DAHW) and the Research Centre Borstel (FZB), also from Germany. It called for the treatment of leprosy using isoprodian—which combined the three anti-tuberculosis agents isoniazid, prothionamide and dapsone—in combination with rifampicin (RMP). A total of 261 individuals, including 201 registered cases of leprosy reported by the health authority of Malta at the time plus patients diagnosed subsequently, proceeded to undergo this treatment for periods from six months to seven years. All patients were reported to have been cured.

A follow-up study was carried out during the 27 years from the MLEP's start, ending in December 1999. From the Maltese side the project had been led by Dr. George Depasquale, who had studied under Professor Griffiths, and prior to our meeting Professor Griffiths had confirmed with the doctor what had subsequently transpired. According to Dr. Depasquale's information, at the time of my visit there were records of around a hundred people still alive who had been treated and cured of leprosy; moreover, no new cases had been reported in the previous six years. As a result of MLEP, Malta has indeed succeeded in eradicating leprosy.

Unfortunately, I was unable to learn how these hundred or so people were doing, or who the last new patients were and what their situation now was. I had heard that when the isolation facilities at St. Bartholomew Hospital and on Gozo were closed, the 22 inmates who had no homes to return to had been relocated to the site of a former army barracks on Malta called Hal-Ferha Estate, where they were provided with places to live and some land to cultivate. They were also said to be receiving pensions and had access to medical care. But when I made enquiries of the health ministry and the Knights of Malta about this prior to my visit, I was unable to receive a definitive answer.

When I asked Professor Griffiths about this, he kindly agreed to accompany me to the site. "Thirty years have already passed, so I don't know what condition it's in," he cautioned me. "But years ago I went there on several occasions, so let's go and take a look."

We left on our exploration in the early evening, as the sun was slowly beginning to set with a golden glow of the kind so typical of Malta. We drove for about twenty minutes through a number of small towns until we came upon a road sign that said "Hal-Ferha". Proceeding further we reached a sector where brown stone walls lined both sides of a narrow, twisting lane. There were no homes to be seen anywhere. All we found were broken stones and scraps of wood; the whole area was overgrown with weeds and bushes. It was then that we noticed a stone in the lower portion of a corner wall painted with the faded words "Hal-Ferha".

And so it was, with the sun now about to slip below the horizon, that we confirmed that the Hal-Ferha Estate no longer existed.

That Malta eliminated leprosy on its own stands as a remarkable achievement. But when I pondered how this history was now fading away, I felt a strong urge to do something.

Even if the day comes when leprosy is eradicated completely from the world, its history should never be forgotten. We have a duty to acknowledge the mistakes that were made in ostracizing people with the disease, as well as the courage of those who endured such treatment.

My visit to Malta made me feel this need all the more.

Culion: from island of despair to island of hope

Culion is an island situated in the north of the Philippines' Palawan Province, approximately 320 kilometres south-west of the country's main island of Luzon. With a land area of some 390 square kilometres, Culion was at one time the world's largest leprosy colony, home to no fewer than seven thousand patients. Culion also had a major impact on the policies toward leprosy adopted by countries in other countries. In Japan, the Nagashima Aiseien leprosarium located on the island of Nagashima in Okayama Prefecture was modelled on the facilities at Culion.

It was the United States that designated Culion as an island where leprosy patients would be isolated, a decision made during the years when the Philippines was an American dependency. An American precedent already existed at the time in the existence of an isolation colony on the island of Molokai in the Hawaiian archipelago. The first contingent of leprosy patients, 370 in all, were brought to Culion, from Cebu Island, on 27 May 1906 under the direction of the Board of Health established in the Philippines by the U.S. authorities. That initial group was met by a mere handful of medical staff, a Jesuit priest and four French sisters of the Order of St. Paul of Chartres. The number of inhabitants grew steadily thereafter at a pace of between 500 and 1,500 new patients per year, who were brought from all regions of the country.

Initially the island was not equipped with a hospital. With staff and pharmaceuticals in short supply, records indicate that up to 1,221 patients died at Culion every year from malaria and other diseases. As a consequence, Culion Island became feared by Filipinos as an island of despair, a land of the living dead.

Culion's high mortality rate continued for many years, and between 1906 and 1980 some 22,000 inhabitants met their death while incarcerated here. Fortunately, as hospital facilities on the island gradually improved, the mortality rate declined. After 1910 inmates were allowed to marry, and in 1916 child-care facilities were created.

Culion Island continued to function as a leprosarium throughout the years of World War II when Japan occupied the Philippines, as well as after the

144

country gained its independence in 1946, whereupon the leprosarium came under the aegis of the new nation's health ministry. It wasn't until 1995 that the history of the Culion leprosarium finally drew to a close. At that time the island was granted regional autonomy and a mayor was elected for the very first time. That first mayor was a person affected by leprosy, Hilarion Guia.

In May 2006 I visited Culion for a second time in my role as the WHO Goodwill Ambassador for Leprosy Elimination. This time my purpose was to attend a ceremony to commemorate the centennial anniversary since the time the first patients were sent into isolation on the island. At the time of my visit, the population was around twenty thousand, of whom there were 158 persons affected by leprosy. There were no longer any cases under treatment. For the rest, the population consisted mainly of descendants of former patients or medical staff and residents who settled in Culion from other islands. From its dark history as an island of despair, modern Culion had been transformed into an island of hope.

The Nippon Foundation, working through the Sasakawa Memorial Health Foundation, has been undertaking activities in support of Culion since 2004: providing small-scale business loans, supplying schools with educational equipment, and so on. Today sanatoriums all around Japan support Culion, and the marker unveiled at the centennial celebration was erected with the cooperation of Nagashima Aiseien.

Nagashima Aiseien and Culion are also connected through music. Culion has a band comprising people affected by leprosy, and Nagashima Aiseien has a similar music group called the Bluebird Band. Koichi Kondo, one of the core members of the Bluebirds, made a presentation to their counterparts in Culion of new instruments and uniforms.

Getting to Culion from Manila involves travelling by plane, car and boat. When I reached the island, I was given a musical welcome at the pier by the Culion Band, decked out in their new uniforms and playing their new instruments.

The broad open space where the commemorative marker was to be unveiled was already a scene of bustling excitement when I arrived. The tiny island's infrastructure was strained to capacity for the occasion, as many people who had relocated to other islands or provinces or even overseas returned to Culion for this special day. I was told that for the previous several days there had been periods when the water supply or electricity was interrupted, causing great havoc. But the day I arrived, both the water and power had been fully restored.

The ceremony began with a re-enactment, by people affected by leprosy, of the arrival of the first batch of leprosy patients to the island a hundred years earlier. Watching scenes depicting how patients had been parted from their families, or scenes of the Catholic sisters and priest welcoming patients being carried in on stretchers, brought tears to many in the audience. The commemorative marker was situated at the spot where those very first inhabitants of Culion had landed on the island. It had been erected in the hope that Culion's history as a leprosy colony—the suffering and sacrifice of patients, the dedicated service of medical staff, and the island's contribution to increasing our knowledge of the disease through research—would never be forgotten.

Following the marker's unveiling, the venue shifted to the Culion Museum and Archives for a ribbon-cutting ceremony to mark the opening of this new facility, funded by the Sasakawa Memorial Health Foundation, presenting Culion's history as a leprosy colony. The ground floor is dedicated to re-creations showing how the leprosarium looked in its earliest days, exhibits of early medical instruments, photographs of patients and the treatments they received. Seeing the enormous size of the syringes that had been used to inject patients with chaulmoogra oil, the only treatment available for leprosy at the time, I was speechless when thinking of the painful conditions leprosy patients had endured in their quest for a cure. The upper floor is home to the Culion archives. When I visited, it was stacked high with assorted boxes of materials, patient medical records and the like, all awaiting proper archiving on microfilm. This archiving work has subsequently been undertaken by experts who volunteered to help with this project.

The bulk of the items on display were collected by Dr. Arturo Cunanan, Jr., the central figure in the project to establish the museum and archives. Dr. Cunanan's grandparents were among the first patients to be sent to Culion, and Dr. Cunanan grew up on the island. Later he won a scholarship enabling him to attend university in Manila, where he proceeded to study medicine. Upon the completion of his degree he had the opportunity to remain and work in Manila, but he chose to return to Culion in order to help the island's residents. In addition to serving as the chief physician at the sanatorium, Dr. Cunanan is a leading force in the drive to revitalize the island. To preserve Culion's heritage, he personally combed the sanatorium, former nursery and other facilities and, virtually singlehandedly, collected and preserved materials that were on the verge of being thrown away, including photos taken in the 1920s and unpublished research findings. With the completion of the new archives, these precious materials can now be passed on safely to future generations.

In my speech marking Culion's centennial anniversary, I spoke of how, along with the brilliant progress that had been made by humankind throughout history, this history had also been marked by numerous mistakes, among the gravest being the way that persons with leprosy were stripped of their dignity and fundamental human rights by being forced into isolation. I also stressed how the stigma and discrimination attendant on leprosy continue to exist all around the world.

At one time there had been a movement to do away with the name Culion, but the people living on the island resolved, bravely and proudly, to keep the name intact—a decision I heartily applaud. As the residents of Culion thus set out to begin the second hundred years of their history, I voiced my hope that the first hundred years in Culion's history would be duly recorded and preserved, and to that end I hoped that the museum would be further improved. The history of this island, I feel, is an important legacy for all humankind.

I became extremely eager for a Global Appeal, with contributions by people affected by leprosy themselves, to be held in the Philippines, the country where, at Culion, people have overcome the stigma and discrimination associated with their disease and started down the path toward a new phase in their history. And so it came about that, as a follow-up to the first Global Appeal held in New Delhi in 2006, I decided that the second Global Appeal would be organized the following year in Manila.

January 2007 thus found me in the Philippines again, this time in Manila in my role as organizer of the second Global Appeal.

The morning of 29 January, the day on which the ceremonies were to take place, as I sat in the restaurant of Manila's Heritage Hotel sipping coffee, I found my emotions rising at the scene around me. The Heritage Hotel is a five-star hotel of long standing that exudes an air of great refinement. And here, in its restaurant, were people affected by leprosy, participants in the scheduled events of the day, eating breakfast just like any other hotel guests. There should be nothing out of the ordinary about this, and yet the scene unfolding before me was a dream I had long held: people affected by leprosy eating breakfast together with the other hotel guests, not separated from them, enabling them to start their new day pleasantly. As I watched what was happening around me, I thought deeply of the long time it had taken for something so inherently normal to actually become normal.

Among the people affected by leprosy having breakfast that morning in the Heritage Hotel were a number from Culion. For not a few of them, the occasion was the first time in their lives they had ever left the island, and the first time they had ever stayed in a hotel.

Several hours later we all—I together with people affected by leprosy who had come from all around the Philippines and countries scattered across the globe—gathered at the Philippine International Convention Center (PICC), where I proclaimed the Global Appeal 2007, calling for the restoration of the dignity of persons affected by leprosy. The appeal, formally advocating an end to the social stigma and discrimination against people affected by leprosy, was signed by 16 leaders representing such people around the world. The Japanese signatory was Michihiro Koh, general secretary of the National Association of Residents of Hansen's Disease Sanatoriums. I also affixed my signature to the document in my position as chairman of the Nippon Foundation.

Global Appeal 2007 addressed the continuing existence, even today, of the stigma and discrimination attached to leprosy—targeting not only those who suffer or once suffered from this disease but also their family members as well. "Denying the inherent human rights of anyone on the basis of disease is indefensible," the document read. "Silence on this issue is not acceptable. We urge you to join us in the fight to end this social injustice."

The ceremony in Manila was attended by more than three hundred individuals, including not only people affected by leprosy but also various persons involved in the WHO. Nick Deocampo, an Asian film historian, gave a presentation on the depictions of leprosy in film. Professor Yozo Yokota, a member of the UN Sub-Commission on the Promotion and Protection of Human Rights, spoke on leprosy as a human rights issue. The Global Appeal manifesto was then read aloud by 11-year-old Ma Kristina Sacdalan, a young girl who contracted leprosy as a child but overcame the disease through multidrug therapy. As she performed her role at the centre of the media's phalanx of cameras, the words she spoke were greeted with warm and enthusiastic applause from the entire audience.

My personal goal is to do everything within my means to realize a society in which, much like the scene I witnessed at breakfast at the Heritage Hotel, people affected by leprosy and their families can travel to any country they wish and eat where they please. This is a dream my father, Ryoichi Sasakawa, was unable to realize during his lifetime, and now realizing such a dream is the mission I have been given.

Through my visit to Culion Island and the subsequent convening of Global Appeal 2007 in Manila, my resolve to achieve a world free of leprosy and the discrimination it causes was renewed. I was inspired by the many people I met who spoke publicly about their experiences as persons affected by leprosy so that this negative legacy of humanity—the prejudice and discrimination they endured at the hands of society—is not allowed to be forgotten. I cannot express my appreciation to them deeply enough.

UNFORGETTABLE PLACES, UNFORGETTABLE FACES

Raibyo-shima: a product of Japanese colonial policy

11 November 2010 found me in the Republic of Palau, a chain of islands that form part of Micronesia, visiting Belau National Hospital in Koror, the archipelago's largest city. It was there that I learned that not far away was a place called Raibyo-shima—meaning "Leprosy Island" in Japanese. I was stunned to discover that here in the South Pacific, so far from Japan, was an island so named. I immediately wanted to know how the island acquired its name, what its history was, and what it is like today.

The main purpose of my visit to Palau was to attend an international conference on improving maritime safety in Micronesia, but in-between events relating to the conference I also made a point of visiting leprosy patients at the country's national hospital. Once I learned of the existence of this intriguingly named Raibyo-shima, I proceeded to make an unplanned journey to learn more about the history of leprosy in this South Pacific outpost.

The Republic of Palau is a nation of some twenty thousand citizens living on islands surrounded by coral reefs and the beautiful waters of the Pacific. After periods when it variously served as a colony of Spain and Germany, and later was ruled first by Japan and then by the United States, Palau gained its independence in 1994. As a legacy of the islands' years under Japanese rule (1914–1944), I was told that the Palauan language today contains more than a thousand words directly derived from Japanese. Regarding Raibyo-shima, I was able to learn that its origins can be traced to the isolation policy enforced by Japan during its rule over the archipelago. I was also informed that as a result of that policy, the people forced to live on Raibyo-shima suffered discrimination to a significant degree.

Immediately after hearing of Raibyo-shima at Belau National Hospital, I arranged for a small boat to take me there. The island is separated from Koror Island by only a mile (1.6 kilometres). As I approached it, not knowing whether it was possible to land there, I was told that the waters surrounding the island were too shallow to approach by boat. Not one to be fazed by such a circumstance, I waded through the ten metres or so of water to the shore, still wearing my shoes. My first discovery was a set of dilapidated wooden stairs covered in leaves and tree branches, which I ascended, taking great care not to break the weak boards beneath my feet. I was sure that this same staircase had in former times been ascended by the leprosy patients who were forced to make their home on this island.

After a climb of no more than ten stairs or so, I found my way blocked by a tangle of overgrown grass and trees—a thick jungle. I proceeded to walk around the area, making my way through vines of ivy and spider webs, searching for traces relating to leprosy; but unfortunately I was unable to find any evidence at all.

After I arrived back at my hotel in Koror, Dr. Victor Yano, the former Minister of Health, who was then serving as Palau's Minister of State for Foreign Affairs, brought me something of great interest relating to Raibyo-shima: a report, 60 pages long, of the island based on investigations carried out by Jolie Liston of the International Archeological Research Institute in 1998.

According to Liston's report, Raibyo-shima's official name is Ngerur Island. The island is 4 acres in area, 350 metres long and 250 metres wide, rising at its highest point to 30 metres above sea level. Formerly a volcano, Ngerur is a geological rarity. Leprosy facilities, consisting of three Japanese-style houses and a well, were established here in 1931. Initially there were 18 patients receiving treatment. Although it is unclear how long the island continued to serve as a leprosy centre, photographs of Ngerur taken in 1998 showed houses where patients once lived as well as graves. Apparently these vestiges remain on the side of the island opposite to where I had landed. I sorely regretted not having seen Liston's report before going to the island.

I was told that a man in his eighties who was a former resident of the leprosy facilities on Raibyo-shima was still living on Koror Island, but unfortunately I didn't have time to go and meet him. From what I was told, he had apparently been confined to the island at the age of 10 and lived there for several years; he was then moved to a different island as the war intensified. According to information from someone who had spoken with this man, a doctor used to visit Raibyo-shima once a month with medicines, and rice and tinned foods were also delivered. The islanders also cultivated their own taro, tapioca and sweet potatoes.

From my visits to isolated places like Culion Island in the Philippines as well as Korea's Sorok Island, South Africa's Robben Island and Indonesia's Bunaken Island, I have witnessed how, in places all around the world, leprosy came to equate with isolation on an island. Of the many islands I have personally visited where leprosy patients were once confined, Palau's Raibyo-shima is the smallest. Possibly it's the smallest such island anywhere in the world.

Through the years I have been driven by the desire to visit as many of these places as possible, to meet with people who have been associated with them, and to record what I have seen. Passing this information on to the world is one of my most important roles in life.

UNFORGETTABLE PLACES, UNFORGETTABLE FACES

Ventures into the "Heart of Darkness": Activities in Africa

Challenges posed by support activities in Africa

A majority of people, both in Japan and elsewhere, probably have a fairly good awareness of the geographic positions of the countries in northern Africa—Egypt, Morocco, Algeria and so on. But when it comes to the regions south of the Sahara Desert—sub-Saharan Africa—few people would be able even to name all the countries located there. More than 80% of all Africans reside in sub-Saharan Africa, and because the vast majority are racially negroid, all of Africa below the Sahara Desert is referred to as "Black Africa". In contrast to northern Africa, where the prevailing religion is Islam, the peoples of the sub-Saharan countries, though to some extent followers of Islam, as a whole primarily embrace Christianity.

Of the 54 countries that presently compose the African continent, I have personally visited most of these situated in the sub-Saharan zone. The purpose of my visits has chiefly been to support the work of leprosy elimination programmes or to improve the productivity of small-scale farming under the Sasakawa Global 2000 initiative. I have been involved in these works in Africa for nearly thirty years, and from my experience I have come to realize that conducting humanitarian activities on this enormous continent is a never-ending test of patience and endurance. The underlying challenge is the ever-fluid political situation in African nations.

Because the task of eliminating leprosy is not easy, I have found myself making repeat visits to countries to encourage them in their efforts. When activities are not being successfully implemented, I go to meet the people in charge and work together to probe where the problem lies and take steps to help rectify the situation and get things back on course. On every visit I have also used the opportunity, by means of the media or in direct contact with local people, to convey the three important messages relating to leprosy: that it is a curable disease, that medicine is available free of charge, and that social discrimination toward leprosy is absolutely unacceptable.

Thankfully, the activities I have carried out in support of leprosy elimination have borne fruit: all 54 nations of Africa eventually achieved elimination as a public health problem, although the small island state of Comoros was unable to sustain it.

That said, there is deep concern that in areas where civil war and changes of government are frequent and ongoing, health management could deteriorate to a point where the number of leprosy cases starts increasing again. As with the Nippon Foundation's projects aiming to improve farming productivity, a level of success has been achieved in countries such as Ghana and Ethiopia, but in places like South Sudan we have been forced to withdraw our support due to a breakdown in security.

At international gatherings to discuss initiatives to support Africa, the situation is always the same. A variety of issues form part of the mix—poverty eradication, human rights issues, improving the position of women—but effective solution strategies and implementation plans always prove elusive. The affected countries, exasperated at these indecisions, rail against the West for its failure to provide adequate support. Meanwhile, participants from the Western countries huddle together in a corner of the assembly hall during coffee breaks and in hushed tones voice their pessimism and frustration. "Nothing ever goes right in Africa," they lament. Indeed, pessimism and frustration are the sentiments of many members who participate in such meetings dealing with African issues.

Whenever I encounter situations of this kind, I am invariably reminded of Joseph Conrad's *Heart of Darkness*.

Heart of Darkness is a novella written by the Polish-born Conrad (1857–1924) based on his own experience as a seafarer. In 1890, aged 33, Conrad was hired by a Belgian trading company to captain a steamer up the Congo River, to explore the Congo's interior and investigate the opportunities for obtaining ivory. The Congo at this time was a possession of the King of the Belgians, and in his eagerness to obtain both ivory and rubber, the king imposed cruel and oppressive rule on the local residents. So severe was the treatment allotted to the natives, the Belgian monarch drew sharp criticism even from the other nations of Europe, nations in which forced labour in managing colonies was a matter of course. In response, in 1908 the Belgian Government purchased the Congo from the king and made it an official colony of the nation.

In *Heart of Darkness* Charles Marlow, whose character is thought to be based on Conrad himself, captains the ship as it sails up the Congo River in search of a Mr. Kurtz, a white man shrouded in mystery. Along the way Marlow has a series of nightmarish encounters.

Kurtz is a "first-class agent" tasked with collecting ivory, but by the locals he is worshipped as a demigod. When Marlow finally finds the elusive agent, Kurtz is gravely ill. Before long he slips away to his death, his final words being "The horror! The horror!"

But just who is this Kurtz, and what is the meaning of those words uttered on his deathbed? Through the years many scholars and readers of an inquisitive bent in the West have been lured to Conrad's masterpiece by all this mystery. Some view *Heart of Darkness* as a tale rife with discrimination toward the local population, a situation reflecting the colonialism of the times. Others view the short novel as a brilliant depiction of the dark side of modern European history.

Not a few film directors over the course of time—luminaries such as Orson Welles, Stanley Kubrick and Francis Ford Coppola—attempted to bring *Heart of Darkness* to the big screen, but all eventually were led to abandon the idea, likely because of the difficulty of trying to deal with such weighty issues. In the case of Coppola, ultimately he shifted the setting to the Vietnam War years in his 1979 film *Apocalypse Now*.

The issues raised by Conrad in *Heart of Darkness* today remain, for the nations of the West, at a level of profundity beyond the comprehension of those such as myself who live outside that sphere of experience. Japan at no time in its history ever possessed a colony in Africa. This is why, I have been told by political leaders and government officials on any number of occasions, the African nations are more open to accepting aid from Japan than from former colonial powers.

Even now, in the twenty-first century, *Heart of Darkness* continues to serve as a metaphor when discussing matters concerning Africa.

African nations indelibly etched in my memory

The sub-Saharan countries of Africa, including the Congo region, are not only frequently racked by warfare; in many cases, accessibility in itself is a logistical challenge. Generally, from Japan two days, if not more, are needed in transit, with a number of plane changes necessary. And then even after arrival, in many of the countries I have visited transportation infrastructure is virtually nonexistent. Compounding these difficulties is the presence, besides leprosy, of a host of infectious diseases such as malaria, dengue fever and, most recently, Ebola.

Miraculously, in all the years of our involvement in these African countries, neither I nor any of the staff from the Nippon Foundation have ever become seriously ill or been injured during our travels.

Given the multiple challenges we have faced owing to this mix of circumstances and situations, my activities in Africa, particularly in the sub-Saharan nations, have left many indelible memories—in Ethiopia, Tanzania, Madagascar, Malawi and Mozambique in East Africa; Mali, Ghana, Guinea, Niger in West Africa; Angola, the Democratic Republic of the Congo, Chad and the Central African Republic in Central Africa; and the Republic of South Africa, Zambia and Lesotho in southern Africa.

In the course of my activities I have met presidents who, in spite of the disease rampant in their country, greeted me, the WHO Goodwill Ambassador for Leprosy Elimination, with a look of suspicion, as if to say, "What on earth have you come *here* for?"

To eliminate leprosy, it's necessary first to change the misguided thinking and knowledge (or lack thereof) of such people in positions of leadership. Luckily, in even the most destitute developing countries, once the person in the top position of authority acquires the correct knowledge and information, he or she quickly manifests outstanding judgement and the power to get things done.

When I visited Tanzania in 2005, I was initially greeted by that country's Health Minister. Over dinner she told me that her father had been a patient of leprosy, an admission whose courage moved me greatly. Later the minister arranged for me to meet President Benjamin Mkapa, who, to my astonishment, said he knew nothing whatsoever about the state of leprosy in his country until he was briefed in preparation for our meeting. "In Tanzania we have an expression, 'to be avoided like leprosy', we use when talking about a situation we want to avoid at all costs," the President told me. "I've used it a lot myself," he said, "but starting tomorrow I'll never use it again." And he gave me his word that he would personally convey to his countrymen the three messages that I had brought to Tanzania: that leprosy is curable, that medication is available free of charge, and that discrimination toward leprosy is unacceptable.

During a visit to Zambia in 2009, the President made no attempt to hide the fact that until I spoke with him in detail about leprosy, he lacked correct knowledge concerning the disease. "Until now," he told me, "whenever I passed our leprosy hospital in my car, out of fear I would always close the car windows and speed past. You say you will be going there tomorrow and will be touching and embracing the patients. I'll watch it on the TV news, and then make a point of going to the hospital too."

In all the countries I have just cited, difficulties were subsequently overcome and they each achieved the leprosy elimination target at the national level.

In all countries, Africa included, I have always made—and kept—a promise that when leprosy elimination was successfully achieved, I would come back to offer my sincere congratulations to the President, Health Minister, and everyone else who gave fully of themselves toward achieving the elimination target.

"Eliminating" leprosy as a public health problem is merely one milestone along the way. Initiatives must continue to be taken to ensure that further efforts against the disease continue, and that steps are taken to achieve the social reintegration of people affected by leprosy and the realization of all their human rights. It is to obtain sustained commitments by local leaders and others involved in the fight against leprosy that I have always returned to celebrate the disease's elimination.

Encounter with "Sasakawa" in the DRC

Undertaking our activities was a challenge throughout the sub-Saharan region, but perhaps nothing remains more indelibly in my mind than my visits to the Democratic Republic of the Congo, which I would like to describe here in detail.

I first set foot in the Democratic Republic of the Congo on 6 August 2005. I should point out that there currently exist "two Congos" in Africa, separated by the Congo River. On the left bank, i.e. the western side, is the Republic of Congo (Brazzaville); on the right bank, i.e. the eastern side, is the Democratic Republic of the Congo. My visit of August 2005 was to the latter, which formerly was a colony of Belgium. For close to thirty years (1971–1997) the country was known as Zaire, following a coup in 1965 that brought to power the autocratic regime of Mobutu Sésé Seko. In 1997 Mobutu was overthrown by forces seeking a democratic government under the leadership of former President Laurent-Désiré Kabila, who quickly changed the country's name back to the Democratic Republic of the Congo, as it had been called between 1965 and 1971.

The DRC, as the country is widely known, has the second-largest land area of the 54 African nations, second only to Algeria. It shares borders with nine countries: the Republic of Congo, Central African Republic, South Sudan, Uganda, Rwanda, Burundi, Tanzania, Zambia and Angola. For many years the DRC has been embroiled in warfare both with its neighbours and internally as well. Factors including ethnic conflict, disputes over rights to rich mineral resources, and military intervention by neighbouring countries have fuelled two "Congo Wars"—occasionally referred to as Africa's first world wars.

In more recent years, despite the conclusion of various peace agreements the DRC has remained highly unstable, marked by fierce clashes between provisional government and anti-government forces in the country's northern and eastern sectors, particularly along the borders with Uganda and Rwanda. When I visited the DRC in 2005, security was being enforced by the presence of United Nations peacekeeping forces as the country geared up for impending presidential and parliamentary elections. The Japanese Ministry of Foreign

Affairs had issued a directive advising all Japanese citizens to leave the country or to postpone all intended visits.

The prevalence rate of leprosy in the DRC at the time was 1.91 per population of 10,000, putting the country among the few that had not yet reached the elimination target. My visit had two aims: to see what actions were being taken for leprosy elimination and determine what problems remained, and to secure ongoing political commitment from the DRC government for elimination.

I arrived in Kinshasa, the capital, in the evening of 6 August and set about my activities early the following morning. To begin, I travelled to Bas-Congo Province to visit the Kivuvu Hospital located in Kivuvu. My mode of transport was a privately chartered minibus; other than air travel, the DRC had no public transportation system to speak of. The road conditions were relatively good, and I arrived in four hours.

Kivuvu Hospital is a regional health centre that originally functioned as a leprosarium. As illnesses other than leprosy can be readily treated in the nearby city of Kimpese, effectively Kivuvu Hospital was providing necessary treatment only to patients with leprosy and related afflictions such as neuritis and eye complications. After spending some time talking with hospitalized patients, offering them words of encouragement, I proceeded to visit a colony of people affected by leprosy not far away, where I observed how they eke out a modest living from agriculture and needlework.

The following day, 8 August, I visited the WHO office in Kinshasa for a briefing on the state of leprosy elimination in the country. I learned that the DRC, with its vast land area, was like a continent in itself; it was also described to me as a "department store of diseases", its list of dreaded illnesses on offer including not only leprosy but also tuberculosis, malaria and AIDS, in addition to such endemic diseases as sleeping sickness and Ebola. Under the circumstances, activities to eliminate leprosy were being carried out on a limited scale only. Activities were especially difficult in rural areas, not to mention in war zones in the country's northern and eastern sectors where the provisional government exercised no control whatsoever.

The WHO's target date for eliminating leprosy in the DRC by the end of 2005 was not impossible, but proactive cooperation from the top echelons of government was indispensable in order to achieve elimination at the very earliest stage possible.

I proceeded to discuss matters with the Health Minister, the Chief Cabinet Secretary and with the DRC's Vice-President, pressing them for a commitment to work for leprosy's elimination and for an end to discrimination against all those affected by the disease. Most notably, the Health Minister voiced his willingness to hold meetings between government officers and the WHO and NGOs, to map out a workable strategy for making more effective use of NGO support, which had been sorely lacking up to that point.

To complement efforts promised by the DRC Government, I arranged for a meeting to be convened at the WHO office involving the Health Minister, officials of the health ministry, NGOs and members of the media, my aim being to spread correct knowledge about leprosy to as many people as possible. The meeting was followed by a press conference at which I made an appeal that the three messages concerning leprosy—that it is curable, that drugs are available for free, and that social discrimination is unacceptable—be conveyed to as many people possible. Virtually all the major local media followed up by reporting not only my visit to the country as the WHO Ambassador for Leprosy Elimination, but also the three messages I had entrusted to them.

After completing my activities in Kinshasa I next headed to Lubumbashi, the capital city of Katanga Province, accompanied by the Health Minister, a presidential advisor, and a representative from the WHO office in Kinshasa. Lubumbashi is the DRC's second-largest city. As in many countries where leprosy is endemic, the DRC has a very low population density and its media and transportation networks are underdeveloped, and as a result there are many places beyond the reach of information that is readily available in the large cities. But no matter how difficult it may be to reach such locations, the need remains to get to those locales where the incidence of leprosy is high and spread the three messages concerning the disease.

Getting to Lubumbashi entailed a flight in a rickety old plane that had likely been manufactured decades earlier. Throughout the flight my fellow passengers, Congolese, who are by nature a cheerful and animated lot, were dead silent—until we landed, whereupon they broke out in thunderous applause.

Lubumbashi, situated some 200 kilometres from the DRC's border with Zambia, is home to 1.4 million of Katanga Province's 4.1 million inhabitants. The city also hosts a UN peacekeeping base, and soldiers in khaki uniforms were a visible presence. Katanga Province is rich in deposits of diamonds, copper, cobalt and uranium, and in former times the uranium produced here was exported via Belgium to the United States, where it was used in the atomic bombs dropped on Hiroshima and Nagasaki. Lubumbashi remained a bustling and vibrant city, and I spotted a good number of brand-new cars made in Japan. The city's major thoroughfares were tree-lined and well maintained, accented here and there by older buildings in the Belgian colonial style.

I began my visit in Lubumbashi with a meeting with Katanga's provincial Governor, Dr. Urbain Kisula Ngoy. I informed him that the prevalence rate of leprosy in his province was quite high—3.94 per population of 10,000—and in view of the lack of adequate measures to combat the disease in Katanga, I asked for his cooperation. After our meeting, Dr. Ngoy and I, together with the Health Minister, gave a press conference in a conference room adjacent to the Governor's office. Together we requested cooperation in activities to eliminate leprosy from the roughly fifty members of the local media in attendance.

At the press conference the Health Minister, speaking in front of the TV cameras, revealed that he has two relatives who had had leprosy—an admission, spoken with quiet frankness, that made a profound impression on me. It took no small measure of courage, in a country where discrimination against leprosy is still rife, to reveal the presence of people affected by leprosy among one's relatives. In order to dislodge misunderstanding of this disease, it is vital for a country's leaders, including those in official positions, to have correct knowledge about leprosy and to take the lead in enlightening the public, and in this respect the Health Minister's statement was of great value to our cause.

Besides Lubumbashi, my activities in Katanga Province also included a visit to Kapolowe, a village some 120 kilometres to the north-west. Along the road to Kapolowe I saw many people on bicycles carrying woven baskets of charcoal to market. Making charcoal requires the burning of vast quantities of trees and is thus an activity highly destructive to the environment, but for many poor people it is the only means they have of supporting themselves. The sight of so much charcoal passing before my eyes made me apprehensive about the future of the DRC, one of Africa's greenest countries.

In Kapolowe I was welcomed by a throng of people singing and dancing in the main square, which is located close to the local leprosy hospital and to a small community of people affected by leprosy. There must have been several hundred people on hand, including leprosy patients, former patients, hospital staff and villagers from surrounding communities. The lingua franca of the DRC is French, but in Kapolowe and the area around it the people mainly speak Swahili. Everywhere in Africa, the locals always love to dance, and here in Kapolowe I joined in, dancing together with the local children and people affected by leprosy, enjoying myself greatly. On occasions like this, where one is unable to converse in the local language, I use dancing as my means of communication.

When the time came for me to deliver my message, it was first translated into French and then from there into Swahili by one of the doctors from

Kapolowe's hospital. I then went on a tour of the wards, greeting each patient with a shake of the hand or a hug. In the community of persons affected by leprosy I was taken to, the residents made sandals or weave baskets. I was told that in one day they can make three or four large baskets, from which they earn the equivalent of about $1—not a bad sum in a country where the average annual income is $100. Nothing brings me greater pleasure than to see people affected by leprosy, eager to be socially rehabilitated, engaging in productive activities so proactively.

During my visit to the DRC, an event took place that drove home my mission once again. I was told that in this country, so distant from Japan, there exists the word "sasakawa", used in the sense of "he who imparts light". Thanks to the long time I have been engaged both in leprosy elimination work and in agricultural support activities, the name Sasakawa is well known in Africa. In fact, I was told some people have been named Sasakawa. Learning that in a country like the DRC the name Sasakawa was regarded as symbolizing hope, I was taken by surprise.

From this, my first visit to the DRC, I came away with renewed determination, a solid pledge, to continue my leprosy elimination activities here, in order to "impart light" to patients, former patients, and everyone involved in local elimination activities, so as to live up to the name Sasakawa.

In the land of Pygmies

Two years later, in November 2007 I paid a follow-up visit to the DRC. The previous year the country held its very first presidential election, in which the incumbent Joseph Kabila had won re-election. Joseph Kabila is the son of Laurent-Désiré Kabila, who became the DRC's first President in 1997 after overthrowing the dictatorial regime of Mobutu Sésé Seko in the First Congo War. When the elder Kabila was assassinated in 2001 Joseph Kabila succeeded to the presidency. In 2007 the DRC was thus finally starting out on the road to becoming a democratic nation, but prior to my visit new fighting had broken out between the DRC and Uganda. This unpredictable situation, compounded by a recent bombing, prompted the Japanese Embassy in the DRC to install bulletproof glass around the ambassador's desk in his office.

To ensure the safety both of myself and of the staff accompanying me to the DRC, a fairly loose schedule was arranged and every measure possible was taken to gather local information. I was fully prepared, if necessary, to change my intended itinerary or to shorten my stay in the country.

As of November 2007 only four nations had not yet achieved the leprosy elimination target: Brazil, Mozambique, Nepal and the DRC. Tanzania had been removed from the list the previous year. According to a report I received from WHO staff active in the DRC, the country was starting to emerge from its long period of civil unrest and a health system was beginning to take shape nationwide, and as a result the leprosy elimination programme was moving forward with increasing impact. In February 2007 a new Health Minister had been appointed, and according to the WHO report he was said to be taking a proactive stance in the campaign to wipe out leprosy.

During my visit I met with the DRC's Prime Minister, Antoine Gizenga. He personally described how in the turmoil of war many of his country's citizens had been forced to leave their homes, a situation that prevented the government from knowing just how many leprosy patients the DRC still had. But he said that after seeing the work I, a foreigner, was doing in his country, he pledged to lend his full support to my activities. I also met with the DRC's Health Minister, Dr. Victor Makwenge Kaput, and he too gave me his word that the government considered public health an issue of utmost importance, and he indicated his strong determination to implement measures to fight leprosy. Granted, promises such as these are in part probably no more than lip service paid to a guest. But I did have the definite impression that both men were sincere in their offers to support our work in their country.

The foremost purpose of this visit to the DRC in November 2007 was to travel to Orientale Province, in the country's north-eastern sector, to investigate the state of leprosy among the local minority forest dwellers, commonly known as Pygmies. Prior to this visit to the DRC, I had been informed that the prevalence rate of leprosy was extremely high among the Pygmies. The north-eastern quarter of the country was still quite dangerous due to lingering skirmishes, but Health Minister Kaput, with authorization from the Prime Minister, agreed to take leave from his parliamentary duties and accompany me for two days to this perilous area of his nation. Meeting up with the Pygmies, who continuously move about within the forests, was thought to be an extremely challenging task—but ultimately we succeeded in our mission.

Pygmies are hunter-gatherers who typically live in the tropical rainforests close to the equator. They can be found throughout Central Africa, and in the DRC they comprise roughly 10% of the population. Pygmies characteristically experience a slowdown in physical growth in their early teens, and even after reaching adulthood their average height is less than 150 centimetres (4 feet 11 inches). This physique is often said to be the result of their adaptation to their environment of dense forests cut off from outside contacts.

From Kinshasa, the DRC's capital, it was a four-hour flight, across 1,600 kilometres, in a 17-seat propeller plane to Kisangani, the capital of Orientale

Province. Orientale has a total land area of 503,239 square kilometres and a population of approximately 8.2 million. Until very recently the province had been the scene of incursions by militia from neighbouring Rwanda, resulting in many deaths, but when I visited, the situation had stabilized and recovery was said to be under way.

From Kisangani our destination—an administrative district called Wamba—was another 600 kilometres to the north-east. This time our mode of transportation was a single-engine Cessna, and we took off from Kisangani not knowing whether the airstrip at Wamba was in a usable state. The plane, piloted by an American, had been chartered from the African Inland Mission, an evangelical Christian mission agency undertaking humanitarian work throughout Africa. It had seating for nine passengers plus the co-pilot, which would have posed no problem except that the provincial Health Minister suddenly decided to accompany us, making for ten passengers. For safety reasons the pilot adamantly refused to allow more than the prescribed number of passengers, so one member of our party, Dr. Landry Bide of the WHO Regional Office for Africa, agreed to stay behind. Once this matter was settled, the pilot crossed himself and said a prayer that we all reach our destination safely.

Our flight was smooth and we reached Wamba in approximately one hour and twenty minutes. From the air I spotted a small open area of red dirt that had been cleared in the middle of the jungle, and in this clearing a large crowd of people awaited our landing. This landing strip had been hastily prepared by the locals over the course of the past several days, literally cut from the jungle surroundings, and at its far end tall trees still remained standing. The pilot, for good reason, was visibly nervous as we made our approach, his face turning quickly from left to right, and back to left, as he gauged our position. We circled around twice before he felt ready to attempt a landing, and our descent was steep and sudden. As we hit the ground, the plane jolted fiercely before finally coming to a stop just within the boundaries of the airstrip.

Our arrival was greeted enthusiastically by hundreds of Pygmies, the level of their excitement raised all the more by the uncommon sight of an aeroplane. Their boisterous clamour contrasted dramatically with the forces on hand to guard us: soldiers, perhaps a dozen in number, dressed in full combat gear including gas masks, plus a good number of police officers, armed with rifles, lining the airstrip from one end to the other. The dire security situation was immediately palpable, yet the Pygmies grew all the more eager in their welcome, singing and dancing at a feverish pitch.

A young girl emerged from the crowd and, with her small hands, offered me a bouquet of flowers. By her side stood her mother holding a small infant—the child of the young girl, I was told. I was completely taken aback at how very young the Pygmies marry, at tender ages unthinkable to us.

From the airstrip we proceeded by car over a bumpy road for some thirty minutes, our vehicle guarded front and rear by the soldiers in full gear. When we reached the heart of the village, once again we were given a wild welcome, this time by nearly five hundred Pygmies who had gathered from their homes in the surrounding forests. Some had travelled on foot over distances of 20 to 30 kilometres to reach Wamba, arriving three days before us in order to practise their dance of welcome and await our arrival.

The Pygmies were all—men and women, young and old—noticeably short in stature. Their bare upper torsos almost invariably showed visible signs of a skin disease of one sort or another: some with the patches characteristic of leprosy, but others with blisters or ulcerations of the kind caused by chickenpox. The sight provided me with ample indication of the harsh lives the Pygmies endure in their forest habitat. I was told that skin diseases are rife among the Pygmies. Among those who had gathered in Wamba, some had deformities of their feet or permanently bent fingers, but I saw virtually no cases of severe disability. Later I learned that only those capable of walking had made the journey; those with severe disabilities had remained back in the forest.

As I walked along shaking hands with each of them, I noted the state of their skin, and some of the Pygmies shook visibly when I touched them.

The Wamba district has a total population of approximately 100,000, including 30,000 Pygmies. I was told that the district's prevalence rate was 57 cases per 10,000, but just how accurate this statistic is, is uncertain.

Being hunter-gatherers, Pygmies move from place to place with the changing of the seasons, never settling down in a permanent domicile, and for this reason keeping track of cases is extremely difficult. I was told that doctors and nurses go deep into the forest on a regular basis looking for leprosy patients, and when they discover any cases they entrust the drugs to the headman of the group concerned. I was also told that the headman is provided with a thorough explanation and instructed on how to manage and distribute the drugs, but according to what a Catholic priest based in Wamba told me, Pygmy society treats all its members equally, and as a result the headman apparently distributes the drugs he receives equally to everyone: both those who are ill and those who are not. This, he said, is one reason why drug treatment has failed to achieve significant results among Pygmy populations.

The same priest also told me that the Wamba area is effectively controlled by people belonging to a Bantu tribe, who are typically quite tall, and the Pygmies labour for them as tenant farmers, a situation that provides them with only a meagre income. The Pygmies subsist largely on food they can gather within the forests: fruit, grasses, small animals, birds, snakes and the like. The Bantu landowners have historically used Pygmies as farm labourers, all the while subjecting them to harsh discrimination. To improve their lot, for the past five years schools have been created for the Pygmies centred on local churches, and at the time of my visit already some five thousand Pygmy children were attending. The priest went on to inform me, with pride, that five teachers had already emerged from among these newly educated Pygmy students.

To be quite frank, I felt mixed emotions at what I was hearing. Pygmies are people who thrive in the forest. They have historically had a way of living uniquely their own: living in the wild, coexisting with forest ecosystems, never causing destruction of the environment, taking only what they need and then moving to another place. I couldn't help asking myself whether it is within the laws of nature to encourage such people to settle down and give them a modern education. Inevitably they would surely become a cog in the wheel of Western capitalism and the money economy, transformed into people intent only on satisfying their material desires. Perhaps allowing Pygmies to live the natural lives they have historically known is their true happiness.

This is a quandary to which I still haven't found a proper answer. In my activities to eliminate leprosy I have visited a wide array of villages home to tribal minorities, and invariably I have come to recognize that no matter how primitive their lifestyle might seem to those of us who live in developed countries, tribal minorities living in those conditions always have intense pride in their culture. I have also come to understand all too well that even when we provide them with medicine, a highly beneficial product of modern civilization, favourable results can never be achieved if we do so in any way that would offend that pride. From such peoples I have learned that instead of imposing on them a relationship between giver and recipient, it is necessary to forge relationships through our hearty acceptance of the hospitality they are capable of offering us.

And yet, witnessing the changes that Pygmies had undergone in Wamba for myself, I couldn't help questioning whether my way of thinking was indeed correct. To find an answer, I should go with them into the forest and do as they do. I should exchange views with them on so many things. Such were my thoughts as the time quickly approached for me to take my leave of them.

As parting presents, the Pygmies offered us two gifts in wooden boxes: a cute little antelope and a mynah bird. I was also given a "lucky cane"—a thin, narrow piece of wood, about 40 centimetres long, prized among the Pygmies. As luck would have it, it was called into service almost immediately.

When I returned to the open area that served as our airstrip, hundreds of Pygmies were on hand again, this time to send us off. Our pilot, however, had a look of worry on his face. He said that before our departure from Kisangani he had been assured that the runway here was at least 1,000 metres long, and he had therefore agreed to undertake the flight. But after landing here he found that the airstrip was actually no more than 650 metres long. He proceeded to inform us that we would be taking off into a headwind, and if we didn't achieve adequate lift he would abort our takeoff. "So don't be too surprised if that happens," he said in a serious tone.

As on the flight in, we were a total of nine passengers in the small Cessna. To achieve adequate power for takeoff, the pilot first manoeuvred the plane down the entire length of the airstrip and then made a quick U-turn before heading at full speed down the bumpy runway. In no time we seemed to be teetering toward the end of the runway and heading directly into the jungle. "Fly!" I found myself whispering in prayer, with my body lifting off the seat without my intending so. "We're doomed," I thought, and then at the very last possible moment the nose of the Cessna lifted and we headed upward. We all broke out into applause—and with a sense of relief we joked that our success was surely due to our having been protected by our newly acquired lucky cane.

Not long after our visit, I received the following email from the priest we had spoken with at the Pygmy village, translated here from the French:

> The man who brought light to Wamba left with words saying "I will be back".
>
> He was a man who did not give many gifts to the people but he poured out his love to all poor Pygmies with his affection and respect.
>
> He is a very modest and shy man but he hugged and encouraged people affected by leprosy among the Pygmies and gently touched the affected skin.
>
> With children he bent down to talk at the same height with them.
>
> He danced with Pygmies to the Tam Tam rhythm.
>
> We would like to thank him from the bottom of our heart for his paying attention to the Pygmies who have been abandoned by society.

Elimination achieved in the DRC: what now lies ahead

Not long after my second visit, in late 2007 the DRC recorded a leprosy prevalence rate of 0.97 cases per 10,000 people at the national level, thereby achieving the WHO's prescribed elimination target.

To be frank, I never expected that the DRC would reach the elimination target so quickly, and so news of this accomplishment took me quite by surprise. From my visits to the DRC I had come to feel to my very core the sheer difficulty of undertaking elimination activities in that country, and reaching the target with such speed was surely due largely to the deep conviction of all those who were involved in this effort directly on the ground. This realization filled me all the more with strong feelings of gratitude and joy.

In August 2008, I paid my third visit to the DRC, spending five days from 12 to 16 August. This time my visit had two purposes: first, to share the joy of having reached the elimination target at the national level with President Kabila, Prime Minister Gizenga and Health Minister Kaput and the many people who had been involved on the ground; and second, to confirm once more the situation in areas of the country where the prevalence rate was still high.

As in many other countries, even after the elimination target has been achieved at the national level, there are often areas at the state or provincial level where leprosy prevalence remains considerably above the target threshold. Having achieved the elimination target at the national level does not allow for elimination activities to be relaxed; early detection and treatment of patients at the sub-national level must be continued. As of August 2008 leprosy prevalence in the DRC was still high in four of the country's eleven provinces: Katanga, Orientale, Équateur and Bandundu. I opted during this visit to go to Katanga Province's Moba district, where the prevalence was 2.01, the highest in the country.

I arrived in Kinshasa, the capital, at seven in the evening of 12 August, having travelled via Paris from my previous destination, Niger. The following morning I visited the WHO office and met with representative Allarangar Yokoude. "Much leprosy work still needs to be done in the DRC," he stated without hesitancy. "During this visit we would like you not only to see what progress has been achieved so far, but also to see what issues remain to be dealt with going forward." I informed Mr. Yokoude that two months earlier, in June, a draft resolution submitted by the Japanese Government, at my suggestion, to the United Nations Human Rights Council (UNHRC) calling for the "elimination of discrimination against persons affected by leprosy and their family members" had been adopted unanimously. I also suggested that from now on, in addition to curing the disease itself, it was also necessary to take special initiatives to promote the social rehabilitation of persons affected by leprosy.

Dr. Kaput, who had accompanied me on my investigation of the Pygmies' situation the previous year, was still the DRC's Health Minister. "Mr. Sasakawa, let's work on this together—until the number of leprosy patients reaches zero," he said with great enthusiasm. "It's my duty, I believe, for my country."

I also met with Nzanga Mobutu, who, as Deputy Prime Minister for Basic Social Needs, ranked third in the DRC's political hierarchy. I conveyed our three messages: that leprosy, if treated early, is completely curable; that medicine is available at no cost; and that discrimination must be rooted out. Nzanga Mobutu is a son of former President Mobutu Sésé Seko, the dictatorial leader who had ruled over the DRC for 32 years, until 1997, when his government was overthrown by Laurent-Désiré Kabila, father of the current President, Joseph Kabila.

It had never occurred to me that I would witness the sons of two former political enemies working side by side like this in the interests of national unity. I had met former President Mobutu once in Tokyo, when he came to attend the state funeral of Emperor Showa in February 1989. I was still wet behind the ears at the time and perhaps somewhat naively said to the President, "We hear that the situation in your country is unstable." To which Mr. Mobutu coyly responded, "Everything's just fine. I brought the guys most likely to rebel against me with me to Japan." Even now I vividly remember how, placing a hand on his trademark leopard-skin hat, he then broke out in a wide grin.

After my meetings with various leaders in Kinshasa, the following day I set out for the Moba district in Katanga Province, where the prevalence rate of leprosy is the highest in the country. I was accompanied by Dr. Kaput and the WHO representative, Mr. Yokoude. We flew to the provincial capital, Lubumbashi, some 2,000 kilometres south-east of Kinshasa. From there we transferred to a 16-seater propeller plane for the 600-kilometre flight north to Moba.

Just before landing I gazed out of the window, and once again our runway was nothing more than an open area of red dirt. Here too, I could see crowds of local people lined up on both sides awaiting our arrival. It crossed my mind that if the plane were to veer even slightly on landing, a major disaster could occur, but those worries proved unnecessary as we landed without incident precisely in the centre of the airstrip, kicking up enormous clouds of dust along the way. Our pilot was a former military officer from Slovakia, and when I thanked him he smiled broadly and tapped on his left arm, as if to say his skill at flying was nothing to worry about.

Our arrival was boisterously greeted by what must have been about a thousand locals. A group of women immediately started singing, followed by a different group, men, who entertained us with an unusual dance in which they wore wooden masks. It was quite a welcome.

As Moba has no facilities for lodging visitors, we put up in a beautiful red-brick church that had been constructed a hundred years ago by members of a Belgian mission, situated within a village of thatch-roofed houses. I was given the pastor's room to use. On the wall was a photo of Pope John Paul II, who was deceased; there was no photo of the current Pontiff, his successor, Pope Benedict XVI. I had no way of knowing whether this unusual circumstance was due to the remoteness of the location or to the personal taste of the pastor himself, but either way I felt this was a bit strange.

My bed was equipped with a mosquito net but the toilet was outdoors. The mosquitoes that transmit malaria (genus *Anopheles*) come out in the morning and evening, and I sprayed my face, hands and feet with mosquito repellent lavishly. But later, when I went to the toilet, it suddenly occurred to me that my rear end was completely exposed and unsprayed—at which point I lost no time getting my business done and covered myself up as quickly as possible.

At 5.30 the next morning I was awakened by the ringing of church bells. I went into the church and, though the priest had yet to appear, some twenty or so worshippers were already quietly at prayer. Outside, I could see small groups of villagers making their way briskly toward the broad clearing where the market took place, chatting among themselves as they carried loads of charcoal or vegetables on their heads. Time flowed at a leisurely pace here, so unlike what we are accustomed to in our big cities.

Dinner was served in the attached convent where the nuns lived. We all were craving a beer, knowing all too well that this was not a place where we would find one, but by a stroke of luck one of the two people serving us, a woman of robust physique, appeared with a bottle for each of us. That beer, drunk in such a remote location, tasted especially good. Watching the efficient manner in which our two servers went about their work, I turned to Dr. Kaput, who was sitting next to me, and asked, "Are those two nuns?" The Health Minister quickly broke out in great laughter. "They're members of Parliament who hail from here. They came back home a week ago to prepare for your visit." At that point he introduced me to the two women, to which my natural response was to bow deeply as we Japanese so often do. I then had our photo taken together, with my arms round their shoulders.

The following morning we boarded a boat from the shore of Lake Tanganyika and journeyed southward for approximately twenty minutes, alighting at Mulunguzi, a small village of some 1,900 inhabitants. Lake Tanganyika is said to be one of the world's oldest lakes, second only to Lake Baikal in Russia. It is widely known for its many unique species of fish and invertebrates, a product of the lake's unique ecosystem.

As at Moba, here too our arrival was greeted by great throngs of villagers. Some stood close to the shore, knee-deep in the lake's water, eager to welcome us. As we stepped ashore, the crowd broke into great applause and the women let out yelps of excitement. We were escorted on foot to the Mulunguzi health centre, all the while accompanied by hordes of villagers who created enormous clouds of dust. In no time at all my hair and face were covered in dust, which I accepted joyfully as a sign of our welcome.

Leprosy had been rife in the area around Mulunguzi since the mid-1980s. According to a study of the almost fourteen thousand people living in the region served by the health centre, new cases were being detected at a rate of 110 a year and the prevalence rate was unusually high, at 25 cases per population of 10,000. I was told that a plan was under way for a joint investigation of the causes behind this anomaly to be carried out by the DRC's health ministry, various NGOs and a group of American researchers.

As so often happened, before leaving Mulunguzi I was invited to join the villagers in dancing and worked up quite a sweat before it was time to take our leave. Our leave-taking was very moving. As I boarded the boat, the villagers—even more numerous than when we had arrived—waded into the lake, yelping excitedly and waving their hands in farewell. They continued doing this until they were but tiny specks far off in the distance—all for this Japanese visitor they might never see again.

After Mulunguzi I next called at the Moba hospital, a large facility with 150 beds. Dr. Kaput's father had once served as a physician here, and Dr. Kaput himself, I was told, had spent part of his childhood in Moba. As elsewhere, I took the occasion to meet with leprosy patients, shaking hands with each of them. Not far from the hospital's main building, several families of affected persons were living. I was told that even though they had been cured of their disease, they were unable to return to their villages because of discrimination and had no choice but to settle where they now were. Any time I meet people in such circumstances, I am always made sorely aware that there is still so much more that needs to be done to demystify the disease.

That evening we flew back to Lubumbashi, where I was to attend a ceremony at which the DRC Government was to issue a formal declaration that leprosy had been eliminated from the country as a public health problem. The event took place in the Katanga Governor's mansion, and many members of the press and TV crews were on hand to cover it. Dr. Kaput, as Health Minister, read out the formal declaration of elimination, and as I listened I was overcome with happiness at being able to be present on this occasion.

After the declaration was read, the media people posed a number of questions to me. Many were fairly rudimentary: "Is leprosy hereditary?"; "Is there a risk of 'catching' leprosy?"; and so on. The gap between the declaration of this disease's elimination and the level of the media's questions brought home all too powerfully the fact that information and advocacy of leprosy are still much needed in the DRC.

While on the one hand remarkable progress had been made in eliminating leprosy in the DRC, a great number of the country's citizens have died from infectious diseases and starvation amid ongoing civil war and political instability. Instances of inhumane acts and violations of human rights, including rape, are reported to be too numerous to calculate.

The DRC is located in the centre of the African continent. It sits at the heart of Africa's only green belt and is blessed with an abundance of natural resources. To me the DRC is the very symbol of Africa and I cannot think of the continent without it

Desire to Help Asia: Activities in Cambodia and Nepal

Traversing minefields in Cambodia

Like Africa, the nations of Asia have experienced great hardships in modern times inflicted by the colonial policies of the Western powers and, in this case, Japan. The Southeast Asia region in particular developed as a way station along the trade routes between China and India, and each country historically possessed its own unique culture. Such was the picture until the region was subjected to the incursions and exploitations of the Western powers, causing Southeast Asia to be left far behind in the global push toward modernization. One of the most egregious cases of course is Vietnam, a country that became the stage for a "proxy war" during the Cold War era, resulting in its being reduced to ashes. In recent years the countries of Southeast Asia, led by Singapore, have undergone phenomenal economic development as they have scored rapid progress in modernization and democratization.

As in Africa, through the years I have visited the nations of Southeast Asia on frequent occasions in my role as the WHO Goodwill Ambassador for

Leprosy Elimination. At times my journeys have taken me into the area's worst danger zones, as when I traversed minefields deep in the interior of Cambodia. What I have learned from these experiences is that, besides initiatives to eliminate leprosy, much additional work yet needs to be done to aid Southeast Asian countries where political stability remains elusive.

Cambodia was one such experience. I was requested, at sudden notice, to provide support for the nation's election process. It all began with a phone call I received from Cambodia in 1993.

The call was from Yasushi Akashi, the Under-Secretary-General of the United Nations, a previous acquaintance. Mr. Akashi at the time was serving as Special Representative of UNTAC, the United Nations Transitional Authority in Cambodia, and he was calling to request my urgent support for that country's impending first national elections. According to Mr. Akashi, the prevailing view was that the election process was likely to fail from a low voter turnout, but he said it was imperative that the elections were carried out successfully, and to ensure their success he was of the opinion that a broadcasting station was required, in order to inform the Cambodian people of the need for the elections and urge them strongly to participate in the voting process. Mr. Akashi proceeded to say that second-hand broadcasting equipment was available in Australia and he was eager to purchase it, but UNTAC lacked a budget it could use at such short notice. He was calling to request that I come up with the 30 million yen (approx. $270,000 at the time) needed in emergency support funds.

Needless to say, I immediately said yes to his request. Ultimately voter turnout for the elections was 90%, far exceeding the pundits' forecasts, and the elections went off with great success, setting the foundation for Cambodia's rebirth.

Hun Sen took office as the country's new Prime Minister, and not long thereafter he visited Japan. I was invited to a breakfast meeting with him, and on that occasion he requested aid to construct a hundred primary schools to improve the education of Cambodia's children. I consented with one condition: that I be responsible for deciding where the schools would be constructed. The Prime Minister, with a puzzled look on his face, asked me where I intended to build the schools. "Mainly in Pailin, the area dominated by Pol Pot," I replied. The Prime Minister still seemed to have doubts, so I proceeded with the following argument.

What's important for Cambodia, I said, was unity among all ethnic peoples in the country. The new government, I suggested, must of course devote itself fully to the task of achieving recovery in and around the capital, Phnom Penh, which had been destroyed during the years of fighting. And I added that as a result it would inevitably be a long, long time before recovery would get under way in the Pailin region, which had been the base from which the anti-government elements had operated. The people of Pailin, however, would surely harbour a grievance if they felt they were being given short shrift in their nation's recovery drive. But, I said, if I, a private citizen, were to go in and construct primary schools in Pailin, the locals would invariably understand that their new Prime Minister had their interests in mind.

Hearing my impassioned argument, Hun Sen was won over, and he consented to my proposal.

That issue settled, I then chartered a Cambodian military helicopter and went to Pailin to determine where the primary schools should be built. The helicopter, being intended for military use, had no seats for passengers, so I had no alternative but to lie down on the floor, a position that offered me an unobstructed view of the Cambodian landscape below, for the entire way. After about an hour we landed in an open clearing. One of my companions began walking toward a spot where he intended to relieve himself, until a voice rang out, "Hey, watch out! There are landmines over there!" I could feel a chill go up my spine. On closer inspection, I then noticed white lines drawn on the ground all around us: warnings of the presence of landmines.

Building primary schools in places like this would be no easy matter, I then realized all too well. Ultimately it took five years to complete the hundred schools I had promised to Hun Sen, but I believe this project was definitely beneficial to Cambodia's democratization process.

I subsequently visited Cambodia any number of times. As might be expected, my visits largely centred on visits to leprosy colonies and activities in support of the social rehabilitation of persons affected by leprosy.

Besides building primary schools and conducting leprosy activities, in Cambodia I also am involved in establishing a nationwide organization of the country's visually challenged, including construction of a headquarters building, as well as the construction of a school of prosthetics. Scholarships have also been extended to several thousand recipients to enable them to undergo the training necessary to teach in Cambodia's schools. In these and other ways I am actively working to support the country's socially disadvantaged.

In 2008 I went to Cambodia to observe the removal of landmines and unexploded ordnance by Japan Mine Action Service (JMAS), a non-profit organization supported by the Nippon Foundation. My purpose was to show our support to the experts—mainly retirees from the Japanese Self-Defence Forces—who undertake this dangerous work; but from what I was told by those involved, it will take another hundred years before all the landmines and unexploded ordnance in Cambodia are safely removed.

Landmine removal, like restoring the human rights of people affected by leprosy, is a task that will take much time to complete.

Nepal, a land where my father shed tears

Besides India, which I described in detail in the preceding chapter, another country in Asia to which I feel a strong emotional attachment as a result of my leprosy elimination activities is Nepal.

In 1979 I accompanied my father on a visit to Nepal's Anandaban Leprosy Hospital. It was here that I witnessed my father, on seeing an old woman resident, take her two disfigured hands in his own and, with tears flowing from his eyes, say to her, "Why did such a sad fate have to befall you?" This was the first time in my life I saw my father shed tears—something he had not done even when he lost a member of his family.

Since then, the leprosy situation in Nepal has undergone considerable change. A country embraced by the Himalaya mountain range, Nepal poses geographical challenges when it comes from moving from one region to another. It has also long been a hotbed of political instability. Yet despite these obstacles, concerted efforts went into promoting an elimination programme to enable patients, no matter where they might be located, to be diagnosed early and given the medicines they require to treat their affliction. In the late 1980s Nepal had a high prevalence rate of 70 cases per 10,000 of the population, but by 2004 the figure had plunged to just 2.4.

Even so, Nepal remained the last country in Asia where the elimination target had yet to be achieved. In particular, the prevalence rate remained high in the country's western mountainous region and in the south-east, along the national border with India. Conducting elimination activities was a challenge fraught with extreme difficulties, exacerbated by a poor security situation.

In response, I have visited Nepal any number of times through the years to encourage the government to extend elimination activities to areas that were not being reached, in order to make a final push toward achieving elimination throughout the country.

In 2004 I visited Kathmandu, the capital, and its surrounding area for a period of four days. During that time I met with Prime Minister Surya Bahadur Thapa, Health Secretary Lokman Singh Karki, and Director-General of the Department of Health Services Dr. B.D. Chataut, among others, and secured a promise to use school curriculums and the media to convey correct knowledge about leprosy to the people of Nepal. Unfortunately I had to forgo conducting any activities in those areas where leprosy was most prevalent owing to a deterioration in the security situation caused by rebel Maoist elements, but I was able to visit the Khokana State Leprosarium outside Kathmandu operated by the Nepal Leprosy Relief Association (NELRA) as well as the Anandaban Leprosy Hospital—where a quarter-century earlier I had seen my father shed tears for the very first time. The Anandaban hospital is also where Dr. Yo Yuasa, executive and medical director of the Sasakawa Memorial Health Foundation, had served as medical superintendent during the 1970s. It is Nepal's largest leprosy hospital, established in 1957 by the Leprosy Mission International of England. It is located 16 kilometres south of Kathmandu in the Lalitpur district, in a valley setting approximately one hour by car from the capital.

Twenty-five years had passed since my father and I had visited the Anandaban hospital, but the facilities my father had donated were still being operated and maintained and serving their intended purpose. The hospital accommodated 115 patients cared for by a staff of 121, and I was told that it fulfils a broad range of functions: from early detection and treatment of leprosy to prevention of disability, reconstructive surgery, rehabilitation of people affected by leprosy, and campaigning on behalf of the disease's elimination.

Among the hospital's patients were people who had travelled from Bihar State in India, across the border. Within this border region, leprosy patients pass back and forth between the two countries, making it very difficult to monitor their numbers and other details, and on hearing this I proposed that a meeting be organized for the relevant parties of Nepal and India to get together and discuss this issue as soon as possible. Another problem in Nepal is that owing to political unrest, leprosy elimination campaigning was at the time restricted to just 25 of the country's 75 districts. A further issue had to do with the fact that leprosy activities, like all social endeavours in Nepal, had traditionally been supported primarily by NGOs, both domestic and foreign. I was told that the country lacked adequate structures to enable such NGOs, which should be at the heart of such activities, to cooperate with their counterparts in the government. Clearly a situation of this kind posed a major impediment to progress in eliminating leprosy, and I keenly felt the need for immediate improvement.

I finished my visit to Nepal with a pledge to visit the country again to the extent that time will allow me. In particular, I was eager to personally observe what the leprosy situation was like away from Kathmandu, so that I could lend my support to effective measures for eliminating leprosy throughout Nepal.

Nepal's changing picture and the path to elimination

By 2006 the situation in Nepal was changing at a fevered pace. In April, the Seven Party Alliance joined forces with the Maoist insurgents and held demonstrations and staged a general strike. In response, by direction of King Gyanendra, Prime Minister Girija Prasad Koirala and other leaders entered into peace talks with the Maoists and preparations moved toward holding elections for installing a national constituent assembly.

By this time the prevalence rate of leprosy in Nepal had fallen to 1.65 per population of 10,000. According to staff at the WHO office in Kathmandu, if progress continued at the current pace, the prospect was that leprosy elimination in Nepal could be achieved in 2007. Before that could be realized, however, the political and social situations would have to stabilize.

On 27 November I was afforded the honour of meeting King Gyanendra in person. I conveyed our message about the curability of leprosy and the fact that medicine was being made available everywhere free of charge, and I also stressed the sad reality that people cured of the disease were still being subjected to social discrimination. King Gyanendra said that his monarchy was well aware of this social stigma, and he said he would give the matter his close attention.

The following day I visited the Anandaban hospital for a third time. Compared to my previous visit two years earlier, the number of in-patients had decreased to 69 and the number of beds had also been reduced. I was informed that in recent years the hospital was also treating patients other than those afflicted with leprosy: for example, general outpatients and patients of the hospital's tuberculosis clinic.

Another reason for visiting Anandaban was to attend the General Assembly of the Nepal chapter of IDEA—the International Association for Integration, Dignity and Economic Advancement—for people affected by leprosy, which was being held at the hospital. The organization's activities in Nepal were somewhat stagnant, I was told, as some former leprosy patients were afraid to speak up out of fear of subjecting themselves to even greater discrimination. I addressed their concerns with the following remarks.

I told them that in January 2006 I had announced what would become an annual Global Appeal to end the stigma and discrimination against people affected by leprosy. I said that five of the world's foremost leaders, including such illustrious Nobel Peace Prize laureates as former U.S. President Jimmy Carter and His Holiness the 14th Dalai Lama, had pledged to work together with people affected by leprosy to combat the social stigma and discrimination they suffered. I added that I would be bringing this issue before the United Nations Human Rights Council, to have that body establish and recommend guidelines for eliminating discrimination of this kind worldwide and improving the situation as it currently existed. I went on to suggest how there are two approaches to dealing with this issue: a top-down approach such as what I had just described, and a bottom-up approach, i.e. a grass-roots effort to take up this issue with the government, which I said was of extreme importance also. And for this to be accomplished, I said it would be necessary to make the Nepal chapter of IDEA stronger. My hope, I told the assembled audience, was that the Nepal chapter would undertake activities that, with cooperation from their government, would let them serve as a model for the entire world, and I expressed my willingness to cooperate with them.

The following day, 29 November, I attended a seminar on leprosy elimination organized by the WHO. It was a two-day affair intended to cover a wide range of topics, including a review of the elimination situation in Nepal and identification of remaining problems; detection and treatment of leprosy patients in the area along the border between Nepal and India; and the role of the media, social service providers and other related groups. The seminar members used the two days to draw up specific action plans and proposals.

On the 30th I flew from Kathmandu to Pokhara, a trip of about one hour, to visit the Green Pastures Hospital and Rehabilitation Centre (GPHRC), a facility created by the International Nepal Fellowship (INF) in 1957 to treat leprosy. The extensive area where GPHRC was located had long been feared by the locals as a place where "evil spirits" resided, and it had been donated for the purpose of building a leprosy hospital. Owing to the facility's gradually declining numbers of leprosy patients in recent years, GPHRC, in addition to treating leprosy, also provided general medical care, nursing care, counselling, reconstructive surgery, occupational therapy and rehabilitation services, and also engaged in research of a more general nature. According to Dr. Iain Craighead, who was then GPHRC's superintendent serving on a voluntary basis, having been assigned from the UK by the INF, at the time of my visit the facility had 82 in-patients, of whom 60% were leprosy patients.

Cooperation from the King, and unexpectedly from the Maoists

My next visit to Nepal was in February 2008. During the first five days of that month, in addition to Kathmandu I visited Chitwan, a district located in the country's south-west. The prevalence rate at the national level by this time was down to 1.2 cases per 10,000 people—very close to the elimination target.

Chitwan lies some 100 kilometres south-west of Kathmandu. The area is famous for Chitwan National Park, a World Heritage site. The region I visited was an apparently peaceful place inhabited by simple people, but during my stay people at the lodge where I was put up told me there had been bombing and rioting incidents close by. Such events occurred frequently in Terai, the region along Nepal's southern border.

Nepal is a socially complex nation, home to more than thirty ethnic minorities including peoples of Indian, Tibetan and Central Asian extraction. Adding to this complexity has been the presence of the Unified Communist Party of Nepal (Maoist) comprising radical elements opposed to the monarchy which ruled Nepal for 240 years. The party gradually gathered strength, enabling it to join the provisional government in 2006 ahead of parliamentary elections, aimed at establishing a constitution, that April. In December 2005 it had already been decided to abolish the monarchy, but the political upheaval was still ongoing. To make matters even more unstable, separate extremist groups were becoming increasingly active in the Terai region. The resulting political turmoil and dire security situation gravely impeded actions to eliminate leprosy within Nepal.

Against this backdrop, on this visit to Chitwan I met with local health workers, called on a leprosy clinic, and paid visits to two health posts in the city of Tandi: the Bakulahar health post and the Bachhauli sub-health post. I enquired whether these outposts had received any specific instructions from the government for achieving the elimination target, but received only ambiguous responses, giving me the impression that there existed a wide gap in determination between the central government and Nepal's outlying regions. I was also told that the area suffered from a shortage of capable staff, as well as a lack of understanding toward leprosy stemming from the conservative thinking that prevails in the rural communities.

Chitwan encompasses six health posts and 31 sub-health posts, and distribution of MDT through these bodies appeared to be going smoothly. I confirmed the availability of MDT at the health and sub-health posts I visited. I was also shown the lesions of individual patients with disabilities, and from what I saw, the medical treatment they were receiving was passable. The Bakulahar health post had 16 patients; the Bachhauli sub-health post, four. As a side note, I will never forget the night I spent in Chitwan. It was mid-winter, and the cold wind that blew through the broken window in my simple lodge that night was chilling to the bone.

When I visited the Bachhauli sub-health post I was met by a very unusual mode of transport: an elephant that had been arranged for my use by the health office and local people. I was hoisted onto this magnificent behemoth's back, three metres off the ground, and proceeded to form part of a grand parade accompanied by local musicians. The journey could not have been more eventful: along the way I caught my head on an electric wire and nearly got electrocuted, and when I alighted from the elephant it was in the process of defecating. On arrival, however, I was greeted by a throng of local people, everyone from young students to elderly residents.

From my observations at the sub-health post, I noticed the conspicuous presence of female health workers who were working as volunteers. Though their own lives were by no means affluent, these workers were very dedicated. For many years they had devoted their energies, without financial recompense, to improving the health of local residents, offering encouragement to both patients and their families. I was told that through the years they had also detected many new leprosy patients. On this tour I was accompanied by Dr. Kan Tun, the WHO representative in Nepal. A report of our findings was submitted to the Minister of Health and Population, Giriraj Mani Pokharel.

On 4 February I met with King Gyanendra. He spoke highly of the way activities were being undertaken in Nepal to eliminate leprosy, and he noted the importance of providing his people with accurate knowledge relating to the disease in order to eliminate the stigma and discrimination against it.

I was fortunate in having a trusty collaborator in my efforts in Nepal: Santa Bir Lama of the Nepal Mountaineering Association, a well-known guide to climbers from Japan. Even when I made the unreasonable request that he help me win cooperation from the Maoists in order for us to provide safety for the conduct of our activities in outlying areas, Mr. Lama showed no hesitation. Without delay he accompanied me to the Maoists' headquarters in Kathmandu, a three-storey building in the narrow back lanes of the city.

The entrance to the building was adorned with red flags and an ostentatious display of large, anachronistic photos of Lenin, Stalin and Mao Zedong. Chandra Prakash Gajurel, the party leader who headed the committee dealing with the Maoists' external affairs, was, to my surprise, a white-haired, amicable gentleman of great learning. He noted that, compared with the former era when leprosy patients were hidden away in shacks, understanding of the disease was now making steady progress. "At times communities refuse to admit foreigners out of wariness of their motives," he said, but he pledged to provide security whenever we required his specific support of any kind, telling me to let him know "at any time".

In these ways, during this trip I succeeded in winning understanding for leprosy elimination activities from the King of Nepal and from the Maoists. I departed from Nepal exhilarated by the knowledge that I could ask for no greater reassurance and support, that we could now proceed to visit areas of the country where elimination work had been lagging.

An all-new Nepal

My next visit to Nepal came toward the end of 2008. Although less than a year had elapsed since my previous visit, Nepal had changed greatly in the interim. In May 2008 the monarchy that had ruled continuously for 240 years was abolished and the country had been reborn as a republic. Only recently had I met with King Gyanendra and won his backing for our elimination activities, but now the political system had changed completely, as had Nepal's top health personnel, so I wanted to lose no time in paying a fourth visit to the country.

On arrival I found Kathmandu under clear skies and not as cold as I had feared. I was met at the airport by an old friend, Dr. Alexander Andjaparidze—I called him "Dr. Alex" for short—the WHO representative in Nepal. Dr. Andjaparidze, who hailed from Georgia in the Caucasus, had just recently served as the WHO's representative in residence in Timor-Leste from 2000 until February 2008, a period of great social upheaval during which he was instrumental in alleviating the dire situation in which the people of that country found themselves. He had assumed his new position in Nepal starting in March, a turn of events I greeted with surprise and joy.

Dr. Andjaparidze gave me a briefing straightaway in the airport lobby. He informed me that of Nepal's 75 districts, leprosy prevalence rates remained above 2 per 10,000 of the population in 11 districts, with the relatively highest statistics recorded in the Terai belt in the country's south, along the border with India. He said that special teams had been formed to undertake intensive activities in the districts where the prevalence rates were especially high, on a trial basis. Then, if that approach proved successful, he intended to expand work of that kind to other districts as well. Dr. Andjaparidze said that he expected the elimination target to be achieved in Nepal at the national level by the end of 2009 but he had one major concern: the extent to which the political and security situation would stabilize to allow his staff to safely undertake their activities in the outlying regions.

Immediately after talking with Dr. Andjaparidze I went to meet with Minister of Health and Population Pokharel. Dr. Pokharel was one of only a few members of the Council of Ministers under the monarchy who retained their positions after the new government was formed in August

2007, and I had met him a number of times at international conferences in Nepal and Geneva. He said that "in the new republic, there should be no place for leprosy," and he stated his clear resolve to achieve elimination in his country in 2009. Dr. Pokharel was supported in his position by two newly appointed deputies, a vivid indication of the changes wrought to Nepal's governing system.

In a further development, to strengthen the country's elimination activities in earnest, just two weeks prior to my arrival Dr. Pokharel had appointed Dr. Garib Das Thakur, a highly skilled and experienced specialist, to serve as chief of the Leprosy Control Division of his ministry's Department of Health Services. The appointment of Dr. Thakur in charge of initiatives on the ground, coupled with Dr. Andjaparidze's robust mobility as a leader and Dr. Pokharel's solid commitment to rid the new Nepal of leprosy, made me hopeful that major results would come of our activities in the very near future.

That same evening I also called on Pushpa Kamal Dahal, the new Prime Minister under the interim government formed to draft a constitution, at his official residence. In Nepal, Mr. Dahal is better known by his sobriquet, "Prachenda". Between 1996 and 2006 he had gone underground as leader of the Maoist rebels seeking to topple the monarchy: a group that evolved into the People's Liberation Army in 2002, taking up arms against the military forces supporting the monarchy. At the time of our meeting, Mr. Dahal, still fresh from his role as the top guerrilla fighter, was now leader of the political party having the largest representation in the interim government, a position that put him in the Prime Minister's seat at the head of a new six-party alliance. His political background aside, Mr. Dahal was highly educated, a university graduate who had for a time been an educator. Perhaps for that reason, he looked perfectly at ease in a business suit and was actually quite soft-spoken. I found it altogether difficult to fathom that this gentleman before me had been the leader of an armed insurgency that is estimated to have resulted in more than 13,000 deaths. At the time, the Maoists were designated a terrorist organization by the United States.

Mr. Dahal pledged to commit his government to eliminating leprosy in his country within the approaching new year of 2009. On my part I gave him my word that when Nepal achieved elimination I would return to celebrate the occasion.

To be frank, though, at that time I was by no means optimistic that leprosy could be so readily eliminated in Nepal. As Prime Minister, Mr. Dahal had a responsibility to maintain agreement among the various parties in his govern-

179

ment's alliance and, in keeping with his pledge to the global community (including acceptance of a United Nations mission to monitor the current ceasefire in place), to enact a new constitution. How to treat the 19,000 members of the People's Liberation Army, the Maoists who had waged a fierce war against government forces during the years of the monarchy, was a source of conflict, however. While the Maoists wanted all the former rebels to be incorporated unconditionally into the national military, the second and third most powerful parties within the six-party alliance vehemently opposed that idea. The issue was the greatest factor destabilizing Mr. Dahal's interim government, and there was widespread speculation that the political situation in Nepal could still change significantly, including the possibility of a return to civil war.

Achievement of elimination

In 2009 Nepal successfully achieved its long-sought goal of eliminating lep-rosy as a public health problem. Early the next year, for four days in January, I kept my promise and visited the country again to help celebrate this momen-tous occasion. By this time, however, Mr. Dahal, to whom I had made that promise, had resigned as the country's Prime Minister.

In January 2009 Mr. Dahal had formed the Unified Communist Party of Nepal (Maoist) from an amalgamation of his Maoists, the Communist Party of Nepal (Unity Centre-Masal) and the People's Front Nepal (Janamorcha Nepal). But conflict with forces opposed to the coalition became increasingly intense, coming to a head in May with Mr. Dahal's Cabinet collapsing and the Prime Minister resigning.

Achieving leprosy elimination in that milieu of political unrest was a very moving turn of events, and its success owed much to the many years of hard work performed by the many people involved, including Nepal's own health ministry and the WHO. Besides recognizing their invaluable contributions, here I would like to make special mention of the cooperation received from the media, especially Dharmendra Jha, president of the Federation of Nepali Journalists (FNJ). In April 2009 Mr. Jha had taken time out of his busy sched-ule to accompany me on a visit to the Terai belt in the country's south. There he gathered together local journalists, and addressing them he had spoken of the responsibility the media should assume in the fight to eliminate leprosy. The media, he told them, must work to disseminate correct knowledge about leprosy, and to eradicate the misinformation that so often hampered early detection of the disease.

A number of NGOs that had long been active in Nepal had of course also contributed greatly to the achievement of the elimination target, among them the Netherlands Leprosy Relief and the Nepal Leprosy Relief Association. Indeed, the achievement of leprosy elimination in Nepal, despite the political upheaval, can be seen as a victory earned through the concerted efforts taken by a full complement of stakeholders.

On this visit I was afforded opportunities to meet with the leaders of Nepal's new 22-party coalition government, President Ram Baran Yadav and Prime Minister Madhav Kumar Nepal. President Yadav spoke of his strong determination to boost his country's leprosy activities. "Sustained efforts are needed", he said, "to reduce the number of patients further." Prime Minister Nepal told me about the Cabinet meeting just recently held, in December, at Kala Patthar, at an altitude above 5,200 metres, to discuss climate change. "We had to change planes a number of times to get to such a high elevation," he related. "Whenever you aim for a high goal, it's necessary to take things in steps. Eliminating leprosy is just the first step. What I want is to bring the number of patients progressively down to zero."

The ceremony to celebrate Nepal's attainment of the elimination target, organized by the Ministry of Health and Population, took place on 19 January. Speeches were presented by Health Minister Umakant Chaudhary, FNJ president Jha, and Krishna Prasad Dhakal, the country representative of the NGO Netherlands Leprosy Relief (NLR).

The next day, the 20th, I went to visit the small town of Panauti in Kavrepalanchok (Kavre) district, about an hour and a half by car from Kathmandu. My visit coincided with Makar Mela, a festival celebrated once every 12 years. A group of dancers, wearing frightening wooden masks representing evil spirits, paraded before me beating an array of percussion instruments. Later I was told that people affected by leprosy were among those participating. A staff member from the WHO's office in Nepal told me that they had been given the opportunity to participate in the festival as dancers as a way of rebuilding their confidence and changing their own perception of themselves and of what they are capable of doing.

Female volunteers working at the local sub-health post also performed a song that is used to raise awareness about leprosy. Songs of that sort, along with staged plays, are an effective means of conveying information in rural areas of Nepal where television and newspapers are inaccessible. The song I heard conveyed the following messages: "If it goes untreated, leprosy causes suffering. Patches on dry skin that don't hurt when you touch or prick them are the most important symptom of leprosy. If you get leprosy, be sure to take the medicine you receive from doctors. Don't think of leprosy as divine punishment."

The political situation in Nepal remained volatile thereafter. Prime Minister Nepal announced his intention to resign, the resulting elections went forward amid chaotic conditions, and Mr. Dahal of the Unified Communist Party of Nepal (Maoist) staged a comeback.

The situation surrounding leprosy, too, notwithstanding the achievement of the elimination target, was by no means resolved. The paths leading up to the famed Swayambhunath Temple in Kathmandu were still thronged with people affected by leprosy begging for alms, just as others had done for decades. It will still be a very long time before the common perception changes in a way that will permit people affected by leprosy to find employment and live dignified lives as members of Nepal's society.

Activities in Brazil

Brazil:"We were asleep"

Other than some small island states, it remains the case that only Brazil has yet to eliminate leprosy as a public health problem at the national level. Needless to say, beginning in 2002, I have visited the country a number of times to see how its efforts against leprosy are proceeding and whether or not MDT is reaching the people who need it.

My visit in 2004 ran from late June into early July, and I used the occasion to monitor the leprosy situation in Chile as well. Even though Brazil and Chile are neighbouring countries on the same continent, what I found were widely different situations surrounding the disease.

Chile itself has virtually no record of leprosy patients existing on its mainland territory, and the only place where they were known to exist is Easter Island, which lies at a distance of 4,000 kilometres far off in the Pacific. Easter Island was home to a leprosy hospital until recent years, and records show that patients existed on the island in small numbers. Some years ago, a survey of the island's population of 3,000 residents revealed the existence of three leprosy patients.

From what I was told, the three patients were all of Polynesian descent. They had gone to Peru and elsewhere as tied labourers, and there they had contracted leprosy, prompting their return to Easter Island. There were also a small number of leprosy patients on the Chile mainland, immigrants from nearby countries, but apparently there were virtually no locals who came down with the disease. According to a prominent Chilean dermatologist, Dr. Juan Honeyman, there are three reasons for this: Chile's temperate climate; the country's distinctive topography—a long, narrow country bordered on one side by the Pacific and on the other by the Andes, effectively creating an insular environment; and immunity in the local population built up through BCG and other vaccination programmes. Somehow I found these explanations less than convincing. Hearsay also suggested the possibility that Chileans possess some sort of racially unique genetic makeup. Either way, it remains a mystery as to why Chile has historically had almost no cases of leprosy.

Brazil, Chile's neighbour, by contrast, has the highest number of cases in the world after India. According to statistics valid at the time of my visit, of the country's 5,500 municipalities, 3,521 or 64%, had registered leprosy cases. The Brazilian government calculated the number of patients nationwide at approximately 80,000, and the prevalence rate at 4.52 per population of 10,000. The disease was thought to be especially rife in the Amazon basin, the country's north and other areas where it is difficult to provide medical services.

At the time of my visit, President Luiz Inácio "Lula" da Silva, head of the reformist government that had taken the reins of power in Brazil in 2003, gave high priority to policies of social justice and those targeting the elimination of economic disparities. He also demonstrated strong interest in eliminating leprosy, as illustrated by his personal visits to patients in leprosy centres, becoming the first Brazilian President to do so in nearly a century. He spoke of his determination to rectify matters. "Brazil could have solved this problem of leprosy long ago," he told me, "but we didn't try hard enough. Now we need to make up for lost time."

I called on President Lula to redouble his government's efforts. The administration that had preceded his had undertaken no organized activities toward eliminating leprosy, and for six years the number of patients and prevalence rate had remained unchanged. What's more, the official figures contained many discrepancies, and the Health Minister himself admitted that the government's statistics were not to be trusted. This lack of reliability in the figures announced by the government was a problem of the first order, and now that the new administration of President Lula had come to that realization, it took the drastic step of releasing some 30 specialists who had sat comfortably in their posts for 22 years. "We were asleep," a senior official in the health ministry confessed.

In contrast, the work performed by NGOs and volunteers during that time had been remarkable. The NGO known as MORHAN (Movement for the Reintegration of People Affected by Hansen's Disease) was especially active.

Established in 1981 by a group led by Francisco Nunes, a leprosy-affected advocate known affectionately as "Bacurau" (nighthawk), MORHAN had set up a nationwide toll-free leprosy helpline called Telehansen. The service was receiving an average of 18,000 calls each year, 47% of which were enquiries concerning diagnostic methods or how to receive medicine to treat the disease. Health centres in Brazil's outlying regions only rarely had resident doctors, and they were forced to rely primarily on routine visits. As a result, even when patients appeared at such centres, all too often they could not be diagnosed or treated because there was no doctor on hand.

Another aspect of note in connection with leprosy in Brazil is the active participation of well-known singers and actors in volunteer work to aid leprosy patients or campaigns to eliminate the disease. For many years Elke Maravilha (1945–2016), one of the country's most popular actresses and singers, visited leprosy colonies to provide help to patients. She also accompanied me during my activities in Brazil.

Elke's life had been anything but ordinary. Born in the Soviet Union to a Russian father and German mother with roots in Mongolia and Azerbaijan, Elke emigrated to Brazil with her parents shortly after the end of World War II. After establishing herself as an actress, besides her professional duties she began visiting leprosy patients on a regular basis. "I was so involved in my activities, my husband at the time asked me if I kissed leprosy patients," she related to me. "'Of course,' I answered, and that was the start of our falling out. So I divorced him!" she said with a laugh. Elke's trademarks were her over-the-knee boots that she sported even in summer, the numerous large rings she wore on her fingers, and her attention-grabbing outfits. Elke was looked upon fondly as a "godmother".

Another Brazilian celebrity who devoted himself vigorously to the campaign to eliminate leprosy is Ney Matogrosso, one of the country's most popular singers. He participated in a televised campaign that was revived after a lapse of twenty years.

It is thanks to people such as Elke Maravilha and Ney Matogrosso, as well as the dedicated efforts made by NGOs such as MORHAN, that government measures to raise awareness of leprosy and give the public information about the disease have received a much-needed boost.

Groping for ways to eliminate leprosy

I next visited Brazil in late February and March 2005. On 27 February I attended a seminar on leprosy and human rights in Rio de Janeiro, and on

1 March I visited a regional health centre and the Curupaiti Colony Hospital in Nova Iguaçu, a municipality not far away.

Nova Iguaçu at the time had the highest leprosy prevalence rate of all municipalities in Rio state, at 5 cases per 10,000 of the population. For a period of two years, however, from 1997 to 1999 the health centre had been closed down for renovations, as a result of which 40% of registered leprosy patients had stopped receiving treatment, creating an issue of grave consequences. I was told that the patients had abandoned their treatment programmes for economic reasons, for fear of side effects and so on, but the foremost reason was a loss of faith in the hospital itself after its long closure. I was told that since its reopening the hospital had made concerted efforts to conduct follow-up studies and provide treatment to the local patients, but from my long experience with such matters I was hesitant to put too much faith in what I was being told.

According to the chief local health officer, he had taken up his post just two months earlier; before that, even the most basic health services had not been available in Nova Iguaçu. The lack of medical services was not limited to leprosy, however, he said, but he added that he was in the process of strengthening cooperative structures between various groups within his district, including the local social welfare bureau, education bureau and NGOs. Even more surprising was the officer's revelation that during the past two years no MDT drugs had been distributed whatsoever, due, he said, to major problems in terms of drug management. Other problems had come to light concerning unaccounted-for expenditures by the health office and illegal selling of drugs that were available. The newly appointed officer made repeated excuses about how he was risking his life, under threat from various quarters involved in such shady dealings, to improve the situation.

Curupaiti was a large colony spread out like a village on a mountain top. Besides the hospital, it contained five neat residential districts, home to people affected by leprosy and their families—approximately 1,400 inhabitants in all at the time I visited. The colony's facilities were already more than fifty years old, and on the surface its residents appeared to be living cheerful and independent lives. Issues awaiting resolution abounded, however: rights of residence, land and home ownership rights among them. These issues had been taken up at the conference in Rio de Janeiro.

The following year, 2006, I paid another visit to Brazil, for nine days from 10 to 18 June. This visit had several aims: to investigate how elimination activities were proceeding, to assess the level of discrimination, and to talk with people engaged in leprosy work about what was needed. In the course

185

of the nine days I spent in Brazil I managed to visit four cities—Rio de Janeiro, Brasilia, Fortaleza and Manaus—and get an overall picture of the issues still remaining.

In Rio de Janeiro I visited Hospital Frei Antonio, which is in the city itself, and then a leprosy colony in Itaborai, about 90 minutes by car in the suburbs.

Hospital Frei Antonio is the oldest leprosy facility in Brazil. It was originally a monastery founded by the Jesuits in 1752 and was active as a leprosy hospital until the 1980s. At the time of my visit there were only four elderly residents remaining. They were being well taken care of, were well dressed and cheerful. Among the four I was especially taken with Lydia, a woman then 91 years of age who had been a resident of the facility since she was 7. "What's most precious to me is that pine tree over there," Lydia told me, pointing to the garden outside. The tree had been planted by her father as a sapling when he left Lydia at the hospital. Now, more than eighty years later, it had grown to giant proportions, standing straight in solitude. When I thought how this tall conifer had reached its enormous size in tandem with the sufferings Lydia had endured during the same long years, I found myself on the verge of tears.

Hospital Frei Antonio was constructed when Brazil was still a Portuguese colony, and the main building, entirely in Baroque style, and the chapel—and even the dining room table—are in the shape of a cross. The interior lends a sense of the institution's history, yet it is kept immaculately clean to provide a pleasant environment to its inmates. On the second floor is a room with a large window fitted with religiously themed stained glass etched with the message "aqui renasce a esperança" (here, hope is reborn). The day I visited coincided with a festival in honour of St. Antonio, and although the hospital was busy with preparations to hold a Mass, the priest in charge kindly showed me around the facility.

Later in the day I next visited the Tavares de Macedo colony in Itaborai, outside Rio proper. The colony had been established by the federal government of Brazil in the 1930s. My arrival was greeted by lively music and people dancing and singing joyfully under streamers in Brazil's national colours, yellow and green. St. Antonio (Anthony), I was told, is the patron saint of marriage, which perhaps accounted for the excitement of everyone on hand for the occasion.

During my visit at Tavares de Macedo I met an old woman whose face was severely deformed. She was also blind and used a wheelchair. I couldn't help wondering how her condition could have been allowed to deteriorate to such a degree in a government-run colony that is equipped with a hospital and nurses. But in spite of her multiple disabilities, the woman told me she had seven grandchildren, two of whom were living together with her and taking care of her.

The Tavares de Macedo colony had some two thousand inhabitants, including 250 people affected by leprosy. Here too, the government provided everything necessary to support the lives of both patients and people affected by leprosy; families were permitted to reside on the premises together; and utilities were provided free of charge. These special privileges, however, tempted people who are in no way affected by leprosy to settle inside the colony, illegally occupying its facilities. Also, although Tavares de Macedo was a government-operated colony, no funds had been paid to support its inhabitants in the past forty years and no one seemed to know where the money had disappeared. When I visited, the colony was receiving subsidies equivalent to upwards of US$15,000 a year, but I was told this money is used for building repairs and the like.

In Brazil, political decisions concerning health issues are made by a 48-member National Health Council. Half of its members are representatives drawn from the civilian population, MORHAN among them. The council makes proposals to the Health Minister based on resolutions it has passed, and it also has health committees in 5,500 municipalities spanning Brazil's 27 states to deal with local public health issues, human rights matters and the like. This cooperative approach by the private and public sectors toward shared goals has proven highly effective.

To illustrate: until a few years ago, the prevalence rate of leprosy in Rio de Janeiro was quite high: 4 per 10,000 of the population. Then the head of the municipal health authority concluded an agreement with MORHAN under which the NGO went into areas of the city where the state government was unable to penetrate and carried out an awareness-raising campaign that enabled Rio to achieve elimination at the municipal level.

After Rio I next visited Brasilia, the federal capital, located about an hour and a half by plane to the north-west. Brasilia is a planned city carved out of the Brazilian wilderness according to a comprehensive design created by Oscar Niemeyer, an architect native to Brazil who is also known for his design of the United Nations Headquarters in New York. In Brasilia I met with Brazil's Health Minister, with the head of the Special Secretariat for Human Rights, and with the senator representing Acre state. On the issue of social support to people affected by leprosy, they informed me that the federal government had admitted its former policy of compulsory isolation of leprosy patients had been a mistake and was now moving toward compensation for those who had been forcibly segregated. They added that what

187

was under consideration was not a one-off payment but rather an ongoing pension programme.

On 13 June, from Brasilia I next went to Fortaleza, the capital of Ceará state, some 2,300 kilometers to the northeast. Brazil has an abundance of attractive coasts, and yet that around Fortaleza clearly stands out as one of the most beautiful and refined.

To begin, I paid a courtesy call on the state health secretary. After that I was scheduled to visit a leprosy colony outside the city, but those plans were thwarted by the fact that on that very day Brazil was playing its first match in the 2006 FIFA World Cup finals taking place in Germany—an event of such great national importance that even Brazil's government offices and banks were closed. The whole country was swept up, the atmosphere wildly festive and hardly conducive to serious work. So in the end we joined in and, from the local beach, we watched Brazil do battle against Croatia. We were worried that, depending on the outcome of that match, schedule for the following day might be affected too; but the ever-powerful Brazilian team won the game— to our great relief.

The next day, 14 June, I again met with the Ceará state Health Secretary, this time for formal discussions. This area of Brazil continues to be rife with discrimination. I was told that the situation is especially serious in the case of children, for if they go to a local health centre and the nature of their illness becomes known, they suffer harsh discrimination at school.

I visited two colonies that day. The first was Antonio Diogo, located in the municipality of Redenção. The leprosy hospital here had originally been established as a convent in 1927. With their ochre walls and red-brick roof, the buildings exuded the warm and gentle atmosphere one might expect to find in the south of Europe. The colony, I was told, was home to 92 people affected by leprosy and 194 of their family members, and when we arrived we were greeted by a large throng of people dancing and singing. The houses surrounding the main convent building were clean and well kept, and each was equipped with the necessary electrical appliances, including a TV and refrigerator. The pots and pans hanging on the walls were also polished to a shine. All in all, the lives of the colony residents seemed relatively comfortable.

After Antonio Diogo, that afternoon I visited the Antonio Justa colony in the municipality of Maracanaú. MORHAN had a branch here, and I spoke with its 66-year-old coordinator, a man affected by leprosy. He told me that, unlike Antonio Diogo, Antonio Justa had formerly been in the charge of nuns who ran it along the strictest of lines. To prevent inhabitants from escaping, the colony was enclosed by a tall barbed-wire fence; and on

188

entering the colony residents were stripped of their normal civil rights and had "lepra"—the Portuguese word for "leprosy"—stamped on their identity card. Leaving the premises without permission after 10 p.m. was strictly forbidden, and if someone broke this rule they would be attacked by the colony's watchdogs and locked away in the colony jail. As a consequence, the man, speaking in an agitated tone, said that Antonio Justa used to be dubbed "the town of the dead".

I was shocked to hear how two colonies in the same region could be so different, but unfortunately the severe way Antonio Justa was managed in earlier days was by no means rare in a global context. Listening to the suffering this man affected by leprosy had endured, related with such anger that he was visibly shaken by his memories, once again I felt to the core of my soul just how frightening prejudice and discrimination are. I couldn't stop thinking about why such discrimination had been visited upon those with leprosy throughout history, and about how we have to work even harder to change the mindsets of those who discriminate.

By the time of my visit, residents of Antonio Justa were free to come and go as they wished, and no longer was the colony under rigid management. The barbed-wire fence around the colony remained in place, however, although its purpose was no longer to prevent patients from leaving the grounds. Nowadays the fence served to keep out illegal intruders from the surrounding "favela" (urban slum), who would otherwise take up residence within the colony in order to enjoy its privileges of free housing and land and subsidized utility costs. Colony residents too, I was told, occasionally resorted to selling their rights to their land or home in order to get money. Times change, new problems emerge; I sometimes wonder if it is the fate of this disease.

From Fortaleza, my next destination was Manaus, the capital of Amazonas state, located in the middle reaches of the Amazon River. Even in a remote place such as this deep in the Amazon region, one finds large numbers of people affected by leprosy.

In Manaus I met with Dr. Maria da Graça Souza Cunha, head of the Alfredo da Matta Foundation (FUAM), an institution supported by the Brazilian government. She and her staff kindly arranged for me to visit the Paricatuba health centre in Iranduba, a jungle town of some 800 inhabitants reached by boat travelling upstream on the Rio Negro, which takes its name ("Black River") from its unusually dark waters that look black from afar.

Manaus originally thrived on its rubber industry. The rubber industry in turn was supported by the labour of Italian immigrants who had made the long journey to Brazil in line with the Brazilian government's proactive immigration policy. In Iranduba, an isolated site some two hours from Manaus, there existed an imposing stone complex that had been built for these Italian workers. Later the complex was converted by the French into a school, and then in 1929 it had become a leprosy sanatorium.

At the time of my visit, the inhabitants of the sanatorium were each receiving a monthly stipend of 350 Brazilian reals from the federal government plus a social welfare payment of 175 reals from the Amazonas state government. Together these figures add up to a reasonable sum, and the house of the couple I visited had a television and refrigerator. The husband was a cheerful, extroverted Brazilian, and in our conversation he made no mention of the tribulations he suffered as a result of his disabilities; rather, he animatedly told how as a young man he had been very popular with the ladies. He also spoke of how blessed he was to have grandchildren and great-grandchildren. Whenever I meet someone like this gentleman, people who remain cheerful despite the hardships they suffered in the past, I am re-energized and refreshed.

On 19 June I paid a visit to another leprosy-affected family living on the banks of the Rio Negro. To reach them I travelled by boat. The family I visited was a leprosy-affected couple who were living with their son, daughter-in-law and grandchildren. Their small cottage, painted blue, was located by the riverside. Inside, hammocks were hanging about and wood-carved pictures adorned the walls. The kitchen and bedroom areas were kept neat, and all in all, aside from the inconvenience of their remote location, the setting was ideal. But the shirt the husband was wearing was in tatters, torn under the armpits.

The couple eked out a living making skewers for cooking meat and fish from wood they gathered in the jungle. It took only 10 seconds to make one skewer, and together they made 4,000 in a day. For every 40 skewers they earned roughly 25 cents, making for a daily income of about US$25. Although there was no guarantee of their earning the same amount every day, they lived a fairly good life, their clothing aside. They even had their own generator.

Talking with them, though, I was surprised to learn how deep-rooted the problem of discrimination was, even in this remote corner of the Amazon. The first to develop leprosy was the father. He received medicine on a regular basis from a nurse who made rounds throughout the area. The next to come down with the disease was the mother. She could have received drugs from the same nurse like her husband, but instead she chose to seek treatment anonymously at a hospital in Manaus. Before long the daughter contracted the disease also, and she opted to do as her mother had. This daughter refused to meet us. As I watched the children innocently playing soccer, I reflected in astonishment that discrimination against leprosy existed even in such a remote and sparsely populated place as the Amazon jungle, forcing those who come down with the disease to conceal their affliction.

Eliminating leprosy in Brazil: a dream still awaited

As a result of these successive visits to Brazil I thought further strides would be made toward eliminating leprosy from the country, but unfortunately for some time thereafter the situation did not make it possible to determine when the elimination target might be achieved. Sensing this deadlock, in November 2008 I decided to make a further visit to Brazil. My main objective was to discuss matters once more with President Lula, to seek his even stronger leadership in the quest to achieve early elimination of leprosy in his country.

First, however, on arrival in Brasilia I called on the offices of an NGO known as GAMAH. GAMAH was founded in 2003 by Marly Araujo, a woman affected by leprosy, and every day some two dozen or so persons affected by leprosy come to the organization's offices and engage in various income-generating activities such as making sandals and drying flowers. Mrs. Araujo originally served as a health worker involved in the treatment of leprosy patients before she herself contracted the disease. She founded GAMAH to fill what she recognized as a need for a place where those affected by leprosy, coping with disability and facing discrimination, could gather.

That afternoon I also paid calls on the local offices of the WHO and the Brazilian Health Ministry. It was in the course of the latter visit that something happened that made me have doubts about Brazil's commitment to eliminating leprosy. In meeting with the person in charge of the government's leprosy programme, in not one instance was any mention of "eliminating" the disease made. Undeniably the Health Ministry was taking steps to promote early detection and treatment of leprosy patients, but it was altogether unclear by what year the ministry expected the total number of patients to decrease to a point that the country would achieve elimination as defined by the WHO. Later I was told that inside the Health Ministry there was a shared understanding not to set "elimination" as a targeted public health issue. The apparent perception was that even if the "elimination" target of fewer than 1 case per 10,000 of the population were achieved, this would be meaningless since new patients would continue to appear. Instead of focusing on elimination, the consensus, especially among physicians specializing in dermatology, seemed to be that what was more important was to undertake accurate diag-

191

nosis, administer MDT where needed, and perform high-quality treatment of the disease.

There is no denying that even when the elimination target is achieved, new patients continue to emerge. And yet, without question, setting "elimination" as a target to work toward is effective in raising the intensity of commitment among those involved. What's more, all around the world I have always stressed that "elimination" is nothing more than a milestone; the ultimate goal is to reduce the number of leprosy patients to as close to zero as possible. That evening I met with President Lula at his office. Also present were Minister of Health José Gomes Temporão, Health Surveillance secretary Dr. Gerson Oliveira Penna, Special Secretary for Human Rights Paulo de Tarso Vannuchi, and others involved in the leprosy issue. Originally scheduled to last only 15 minutes, our meeting lengthened to half an hour. During that time I appealed to President Lula to bring improvement to the current situation of his country's people affected by leprosy, and my words were echoed by similar appeals from the national coordinator of MORHAN, Artur Custódio, and people affected by leprosy from across the country.

Although Brazil has yet to achieve the elimination target, this fact should not be interpreted as a reflection of any lack of interest in the issue on the part of President Lula during his presidency. On the contrary, the President was extremely cooperative in the quest to achieve elimination: immediately after he took office, he paid visits to leprosy facilities, and he also took the decision to pay financial compensation to people affected by leprosy who had suffered under Brazil's isolation policy in force through the 1960s. Also, in 2006, President Lula had proclaimed his support for improving the situation of people affected by leprosy in Brazil and restoring their dignity, as a signatory to that year's Global Appeal. During our meeting the President asked Health Minister Temporão for an explanation of the situation regarding leprosy, and he gave me his word that he would cooperate in every way possible.

This meeting with President Lula quickly produced two major results. First, it was decided that in January 2009, when the central government announced the new year's prime objectives to the country's municipal leaders, highest priority was accorded to leprosy as a public health issue, alongside measures to combat dengue fever. Second, President Lula decided to call on the Ministry of Health to send written appeals to the nation's municipal leaders at all levels asking for their help in resolving the leprosy issue. That these major initiatives were determined within 24 hours of my meeting with President Lula demonstrates the strong commitment of his government toward eliminating leprosy.

In spite of my renewed hopes, achievement of the elimination target in Brazil remained elusive thereafter. What's more, contacts made with the Brazilian Ministry of Health failed to provide a clear picture of how the situation was unfolding.

Just as leprosy was on the verge of being eliminated as a public health problem worldwide, I did not wish to see Brazil fall by the wayside. Using every available route at my disposal, including MORHAN, I called for the resumption of full-scale elimination activities by the Brazilian Health Ministry.

In 2011, a presidential election resulted in the administration of President Lula being succeeded by Brazil's first female President, Dilma Vana Rousseff. I couldn't help wondering whether the leprosy initiatives introduced by President Lula would be successfully carried on by his successor. Indeed, the matter weighed heavily on my mind.

In November 2011 I had my much-awaited opportunity to visit Brazil once again. The occasion was to attend the International Leprosy Association's Regional Congress of the Americas, which was being held jointly with the 12th Brazilian Leprosy Congress, in the city of Maceió, capital of Alagoas state in Brazil's north-east coastal region.

During the course of the events a video message was presented of Dr. Jarbas Barbosa da Silva, Jr., secretary of Health Surveillance at the Ministry of Health. A good friend of long standing, Dr. Barbosa is both a man of his word and a man of action. In his message he stated that elimination of leprosy is an urgent issue to which every effort was being devoted, and he expressed his hope that government authorities, medical personnel, NGOs, organizations of people affected by leprosy and civic organizations would work together toward achieving elimination not only at the national level but also at the state and municipal levels throughout the country.

The following day I paid a visit to the Oliveira Santana Rehabilitation Centre, where I observed how persons with disabilities, including those affected by leprosy, were undergoing vocational training. After lunch I then returned to São Paulo for a meeting with representatives of the World Medical Association (WMA) to discuss Global Appeal 2012. After that, I continued on to Rio de Janeiro to take part in an event, organized by MORHAN, where parents were reunited with their children who had been taken from them in line with Brazil's earlier isolation policy.

Legislation requiring the isolation of leprosy patients had been enacted in Brazil during the 1930s, and it remained in force until 1962. In 2007 President Lula signed a bill to provide monetary compensation to people affected by leprosy who had suffered from the past policy of compulsory isolation. A figure central to the passage of this bill was Artur Custódio, MORHAN's national coordinator, a man who, for the sake of people affected by leprosy, would go anywhere he thought necessary: from the President's Office to the depths of the Amazon jungle. Artur is a good friend, and he offers to make arrangements for me every time I visit Brazil.

When the leprosy isolation policy was in force, patients were forbidden to take their own children with them to their isolation facility. Children of young age were in many cases placed in orphanages and stripped of the liberty to ever see their parents again. MORHAN was now undertaking activities all around Brazil to reunite such children with their parents. The event I attended on this occasion was held in Tavares de Macedo, a former hospital colony where many people affected by leprosy still reside. The open plaza where the event took place was filled with an estimated 500 people—people affected by leprosy and children—from Rio de Janeiro, São Paulo and other states. Besides providing a venue for reunions between parents and children, the event also served as a forum for participants to describe the misery of their individual experiences, in the hope that their testimony would arouse greater interest in the issue of separation under former leprosy laws and also give impetus to devising systems to support children who remained alone without parents.

In Brazil, MORHAN has played a proactive role in bringing the situation of those who were affected by former isolation policies to the attention of members of the government and the media. I left Rio de Janeiro feeling assured that with MORHAN this matter was in the best of hands, and I prayed that further progress would be made to resolve all issues still awaiting attention.

In Brasilia I met with Dr. Diego Victoria Mejia at the WHO's country office. We discussed how President Rousseff, who took office in January that year, had pledged to make leprosy one of her administration's most important issues, and I expressed the hope that Brazil would make every effort to locate leprosy patients at the regional and local levels.

Next I went to the Ministry of Health to meet with the current minister, Dr. Alexandre Padilha. Dr. Padilha already knew that I was involved in the issue of leprosy and associated discrimination and that I had just participated in the reunions in Rio de Janeiro between parents and children separated under the isolation policy, and he expressed his pleasure in knowing that I had such strong interest in human rights issues in Brazil. He agreed to take part in the launch event for the next Global Appeal scheduled to take place in São Paulo in January 2012 and the human rights symposium that would follow in Rio.

My final meeting in Brazil was with Ramais de Castro Silveira, executive secretary of the Special Secretariat for Human Rights (SDH), which is directly attached to the Office of the President. The SDH had taken up leprosy and related human rights issues, and Mr. Silveira had a good understanding of the resolutions concerning leprosy adopted by the United Nations. He too stated that President Rousseff considered human rights issues one of the most crucial topics of her political agenda, and he personally thanked me for the work I was doing as the WHO's Goodwill Ambassador. "Discrimination against people affected by leprosy is a violation of their human rights," he said. He added that he would by all means attend the forthcoming Global Appeal and the International Symposium on Leprosy and Human Rights, and he offered to cooperate in every way possible to ensure the success of those events.

After this visit to Brazil, covering four cities with little time to spare, I returned to Japan feeling confident that the elimination of leprosy in Brazil would soon be achieved.

The new Global Appeal was launched in São Paulo at the end of January 2012. The event was organized with the cooperation of the World Medical Association, in particular with the strong support of the WMA's president, Dr. José Luiz Gomes do Amaral, who was based in the city.

The following month, the first in a series of five regional symposiums on leprosy and human rights, which I discussed in Chapter 1, was held in Rio de Janeiro to promote the UN resolution on the elimination of discrimination against person affected by leprosy and their family members and its accompanying principles and guidelines. It was a good start to the series of symposiums, which helped to lay the ground for further work toward ending stigma and discrimination against leprosy in the world.

But although I have been back to Brazil since, it remains the case that the country has yet to achieve the elimination of leprosy as a public health problem. In 2017, the reported prevalence of leprosy was 1.3 per 10,000 of the population at the national level.

I do not underestimate the challenges that Brazil faces. It is a vast country and has a decentralized health system, under which a high degree of autonomy devolves to the 26 states and more than 5,500 municipalities. Hence the commitment shown by the federal government to tackle leprosy may not always filter down to the regions, where issues of infrastructure, human resources and funding exist.

But I continue to have faith that Brazil will one day join other countries in eliminating leprosy as a public health problem, and I look forward to that day.

5

ENCOUNTERS WITH RELIGIOUS LEADERS

His Holiness the 14th Dalai Lama and Leprosy

His Holiness the Dalai Lama and Forum 2000

I first made the acquaintance of His Holiness the 14th Dalai Lama, supreme leader of Tibetan Buddhism and Nobel Peace Prize laureate, in 1997 at the Forum 2000 conference.

On nearly every occasion that the Dalai Lama attended a Forum 2000 conference, I took the opportunity to engage His Holiness in a discussion. Even now I recall his kind words to me when we first met: "I went to Japan for the first time in 1967," he enthusiastically related. "Japan at that time already was a country which had achieved materialistic development and was very rich. Japan has rich traditions and Buddhism is widely practised. I think Japan, with its coexistence of materialistic richness and spiritual values, can contribute more than any other country to the enrichment of human values and the realization of spiritual development."

Subsequent to that first meeting, whenever I have had occasion to talk with His Holiness, I have always spoken of how I consider the elimination of leprosy to be my life's mission, and I have reported on my ongoing activities to eradicate not only leprosy as a physical ailment but also the discrimination towards it, to restore the dignity of people affected by leprosy in India and around the world, to achieve their social rehabilitation and improve their lives. And His Holiness has always responded with a gentle and benevolent look, taking my hand and enveloping it in his own warm hands. Moreover, each time we have met, His Holiness has always placed a khata, the Tibetan scarf of pure white silk presented as a sign of respect, around my neck, offering up a prayer that I might carry out my activities in good health.

On one occasion, His Holiness asked me if I knew Baba Amte.[1] "Baba Amte devoted his life to leprosy and the disabled," he related. "I stayed at the shelter he created for people affected by leprosy, and donated part of my Nobel Prize money to it." I replied by telling His Holiness that I was engaged in work to eliminate leprosy and eliminate discrimination toward the disease. "My hope is to reduce to zero the number of people affected by leprosy who must resort to begging." "That will be difficult," he responded, whereupon I said, "Whether it's possible or not, I'll never know unless I give it a try—and I'm determined to succeed. I give you my word."

Since that time, His Holiness has always cooperated in my activities. In 2006 he was one of the first to sign his name to the Global Appeal to End Stigma and Discrimination against People Affected by Leprosy, the programme I launched that year with support from global leaders, Nobel Peace Prize laureates and many other eminent individuals. Other signatories who had attended Forum 2000 conferences included former U.S. President Jimmy Carter, former President of Ireland Mary Robinson, Elie Wiesel, former Costa Rican President Oscar Arias Sánchez, former Nigerian President Olusegun Obasanjo, and President Václav Havel. Signatories who had never participated in a Forum 2000 event were former Indian President R. Venkataraman and Brazilian President Luiz Inácio Lula da Silva.

Visit to the Dalai Lama in Dharamsala

Having got to know His Holiness on these close terms through the years, in August 2012 I paid a visit to Dharamsala, the city in northern India's Himachal Pradesh state where the Dalai Lama's residence and the headquarters of his Tibetan Government in Exile—officially known as the Central Tibetan Administration—are located.

The name Dharamsala derives from Hindi words variously translated as "religious sanctuary" and "spiritual dwelling", i.e. a holy place. His Holiness the 14th Dalai Lama took up residence here in 1959 after fleeing from Tibet. The buildings of Dharamsala cling to steep mountain slopes at an average elevation of 1,400 metres, standing cheek by jowl, and supporting the lives of some six thousand Tibetans. As I approached this headquarters of the Tibetan Government in Exile from the nearest airport, I was struck by the beauty of the lush green mountains and crystal clear streams. Himachal

---

[1] At the introduction of His Holiness, I visited Baba Amte in 2007. I discuss this in detail in Chapter 3.

Pradesh isn't home to large numbers of people affected by leprosy, and although in my many visits to India I had already been to almost all of its 28 states and seven union territories, this was my first time in Himachal Pradesh.

I began my time in Dharamsala with a nearby visit to Palampur, a village said to contain the only colony of people affected by leprosy in this region. The colony had been established by Christian missionaries in 1917, and I was told that from an earlier peak of around 30 households it now was home to 17 households, including some people who had moved here from Tibet to be near His Holiness. It was a most pleasant environment to live in, set amid beautiful trees. Apparently the colony receives support from both the Christian missionary organization and the Tibetan Government in Exile, and from what I was told the residents have a wonderful life here, totally free from discrimination.

The following day I went to the building that houses the Central Tibetan Administration for an audience with His Holiness. After passing through a rigorous security check, I was led to a waiting room. An endless stream of people were waiting to see His Holiness, and it was nearly one and a half hours later that I was ushered in to see him. As always, he greeted me with an eager, enveloping handshake and warm smile.

"About twenty years ago," His Holiness began, "I visited Odisha together with my elder brother, and at that time there were 500,000 leprosy patients there. I spoke of the matter with my brother, and we wanted to do something for those people, but as they numbered half a million there were too many for us to be able to do anything. That so many leprosy patients have now been cured is truly wonderful, and I want to express my great respect to you and to everyone else who has addressed this problem through the years. When it comes to the problem of discrimination, however, this is something that dies hard and defies easy elimination. In this regard, much still needs to be done."

After a pause, His Holiness continued. "Even after leprosy patients have been cured of their disease, they continue to suffer discrimination. This is unacceptable. Social behaviour and attitudes have to be changed. Religious leaders such as myself, we have to appeal to society's benevolence. Ostracizing people from society cannot be allowed. Instead of shutting them out, society should accept them, warmly."

I then explained how in India there are still more than 800 leprosy colonies in existence, and how people affected by leprosy and their families are all forced to live in isolation from society. Hearing this, His Holiness said he would like to accompany me in visiting a colony some day. He added that we should have the media come along, too, so that this issue would become broadly known, as a way of raising people's awareness. This was more than I could ever have dreamed of, and I felt both buoyed and encouraged.

My original purpose in visiting Dharamsala had been to receive a message from the Dalai Lama urging people the world over to stop discriminating against leprosy. His Holiness gladly agreed to my request, and his message was recorded on video. Here is what he said in full:

Words from His Holiness the Dalai Lama (recorded on 27 August 2012)

Indeed, I am very very happy meeting with my long-time friend, Mr. Sasakawa. Not only my friend, but this person is really taking serious care of unfortunate people, in this case, people who have leprosy, leprosy patients. For several years, he has really achieved a lot of things in this field. Millions and millions of people who had this disease are already cured. His aim is to eliminate this disease completely from this Earth, this planet. Now I appreciate all his work, all those people who are really caring.

Then I notice, after completely cured scientifically, there still are some cases that people are uneasily accepted as members of society. This habit, I think, must change after all.

Seven billion human beings are essentially brothers and sisters. We're born the same. We die the same. Everyone wants a happy life, and everyone has a right to achieve a happy life. Then, we are a social animal. Each individual maximizes happiness, remaining within the society as a member of a community, and shares the common sense of community. That's immensely important. Even an animal, they have no intelligence or education, but as a social animal, when they live together, they must be happier. Any social animal, if one single being is separated from the main community of a group, it's unhappy. So, we human beings are also like that.

Therefore, medically there is no danger to get this disease because they're completely cured. Then, there's no reason. Bring together in the society, share, live together as your own family member. I think really that for human beings, and spiritually speaking also, that's an act of compassion. We pray to God, pray to Buddha, and are supposed to always talk compassion, love, and these things. This is life. Unnecessary discrimination is against what we believe. Therefore, even for a non-believer, as a member of the seven billion human society, you must reach out to every human being. And as believers, of course, we believe in the practice of love and compassion. So we must implement these things.

Therefore, these completely cured patients must all be brought into the human society as a normal human being. That's I think very very important. A believer does great services to Buddha and God. At a human level, I think it is a really important practice of secular ethics.

When I met Indian Prime Minister Manmohan Singh in 2005, the first thing he had said to me was, "Mr. Sasakawa, you have been an inspiration to India." At the time, I didn't quite understand what he meant. Later, I learned that he meant that, for India, I had served as a motivating force. I was deeply humbled, feeling that I wasn't deserving of such kind words. But it was on meeting with His Holiness the Dalai Lama in Dharamsala and speaking with him that I came to know what true inspiration is—and at that point I finally understood what the Prime Minister had meant. The inspiration I might bring to India is of course only small. Real inspiration, I now understood, was the path set out by His Holiness as a person of religion, his empathy for the difficult lives of people affected by leprosy, his words that as human beings we are in essence all brothers and sisters.

His Holiness visits a colony

After taking leave of His Holiness in Dharamsala, I immediately went to Delhi and met with Vagavathali Narsappa, chairman of the Association of People Affected by Leprosy (APAL), to arrange for His Holiness to visit a colony. The visit ultimately took place on 20 March 2014. The location chosen was Kasturba Gram Kusht Ashram, a large leprosy colony located in Tahirpur, on the outskirts of Delhi. This was the colony of Sarat Kumar Dutta, who until his death in 2013 was a leader of persons affected by leprosy in whom I had placed great trust. I had visited the colony myself on several occasions, to see how he was getting on.

His Holiness's visit generated great excitement, for it was the first time a person of such importance had ever visited the colony. Dr. Vineeta Shankar of the Sasakawa-India Leprosy Foundation (S-ILF), who was charged with seeing that His Holiness's visit went smoothly, was at pains to ensure all went off well.

Amid heavy police protection, the car carrying His Holiness entered the colony, where throngs had gathered in eager anticipation. After a brief greeting in my direction, His Holiness proceeded directly to where the residents were seated in neat rows. As he walked among them, he greeted each in turn, taking their gnarled hands in his own. Together we then took to the stage.

I opened with a brief greeting, after which His Holiness offered the following remarks. With his beatific smile and unmistakable aura, he instantly charmed everyone.

I am very happy to be with you here today, as a brother. I have visited Baba Amte's shelter, and I was greatly moved by the joy and smiles I saw there on the faces of the leprosy patients as they all eagerly performed jobs they are capable of, with confidence.

I don't like it when people—even those who have wealth or high position and good health—have no smile. A smile, more than anything, is a sign of friendship.

Even if you have physical problems, you should not lose hope. What's most important is to have faith in yourself. If possible, you should do some form of handiwork. At Baba Amte's shelter everyone performed some kind of job.

Seven billion human beings are all equal. Everyone wants to be happy. People should not look down on others. No one wants to suffer. Everyone has a right to seek happiness. No one should discriminate. Regardless of caste, regardless of religion, regardless of social background, discrimination is a sin. Prejudice must be eliminated through education.

First, you yourselves must strive to have self-confidence and courage.

After his remarks, His Holiness resumed greeting and holding the hands of the many people affected by leprosy gathered for this occasion, offering them his encouragement. He shook the hands not only of the elderly who extended theirs, but also warmly took those of children in his own. He also responded to numerous requests for photos before taking his leave.

The Dalai Lama is known around the world and has millions of followers on his Facebook page. For me, as one who has long fought to eliminate leprosy and address human rights issues related to this disease, the way His Holiness's visit to the colony at Tahirpur made known worldwide the situation of people affected by leprosy and their families was deeply moving. It is a day that will forever remain etched in my memory.

Dalai Lama-Sasakawa Scholarship

During his visit to Tahirpur, His Holiness pledged that he would donate royalties from his writings for the benefit of children of people affected by leprosy. I suggested to His Holiness that, based on his donation, a scholarship system be created that would provide such children living in colonies with opportunities to receive higher education. His Holiness was pleased with my proposal and, with further assistance from the Nippon Foundation, the Dalai Lama-Sasakawa Scholarship programme was launched in 2015 within the Sasakawa-India Leprosy Foundation.

Under this programme, outstanding students selected from among young people living in colonies are provided with tuition fees and living expenses necessary to enable them to attend vocational schools or universities. In the programme's first two years, a total of 29 students received scholarships. After graduation, they aim to work as nurses, engineers, lawyers and in business. What His Holiness and I hope is that these young people, following completion of their studies, will take an interest in, and contribute to, activities to improve the lives of inhabitants of the colonies. Our ultimate wish is that the colonies themselves will cease to exist, that their inhabitants will integrate completely into society.

Making the acquaintance of His Holiness the Dalai Lama has instilled great courage in me. Today, the scholarship programme carrying out his will continues. Something he said to me in particular remains deep in my heart: "Religious leaders must encourage society to be warm and understanding toward people affected by leprosy. There must not be outcasts. Society, rather than rejecting them, must embrace them." I am firmly resolved to continue my work until the day I have fulfilled my pledge to His Holiness and realized my dream of no more begging in India because of leprosy.

Collaboration with the Catholic Church

Through the years, on several occasions, my father and I have both been blessed with opportunities to have an audience with the Pope, leader of the worldwide Catholic Church, to speak with him about the global leprosy situation, and report on our activities to eliminate this disease.

In the first such audience, which took place at the Vatican in Rome in 1983, I accompanied my father, Ryoichi Sasakawa, to a private meeting with Pope John Paul II. His Holiness towered over my father and embraced him. The next occasion, in 2002, I met the Pope at the time of a Papal Mass. On each occasion, Pope John Paul II listened to us patiently, with great sincerity, blessing us and offering up his prayers for the success of our activities to eliminate leprosy.

In addition, on World Leprosy Day, which is observed every year in late January, the Pontifical Council for Health Care Workers—the Vatican equivalent of a health ministry—invariably issued a message of salvation and blessing.

With the accession of Pope Francis, the first pontiff born in Latin America, there have been times when, in his enthusiasm for breaking with the Vatican's antiquated ways, some of his statements have proved hurtful to persons affected by leprosy. In June 2013, at a meeting of the Pontifical Ecclesiastical Academy at the Vatican, Pope Francis admonished the participants for their zealous pursuit of ambition, of personal aims, stating, "your priority should be the loftier good of the Gospel cause and the accomplishment of the mission that will be entrusted to you … Careerism is a form of leprosy, a leprosy. No careerism, please."

I found this use of leprosy by the Pope as a metaphor for something undesirable truly regrettable. On behalf of all people affected by leprosy, I lost no time in writing to the Pope to express my dismay. Two weeks later I received a reply from the Pope's representative informing me that my letter had been received. But as to whether the Pope himself actually read my letter, nothing was mentioned and my doubts remained. Not long afterward, in October 2013, Pope Francis once again spoke of leprosy as a metaphor for something bad. In an interview with the Italian press, he made the comment that in the past, heads of the Church "have often been narcissists, flattered and thrilled by their courtiers", whereupon he added, "The court is the leprosy of the papacy." Once again I quickly sent off a letter of protest. Then, in July of the following year, in another newspaper interview, this time addressing the issue of sexual abuse of minors by members of the clergy, Pope Francis was quoted as calling the Church sex abuse scandal a "leprosy in our house". Immediately, I sent off yet another letter.

Eventually I received cordial acknowledgement of all three of my letters, but I felt His Holiness had never read them. It was then that we decided to take the initiative and propose to the Vatican that we co-host an international conference on leprosy. The task of realizing this idea fell to Nippon Foundation executive director Tatsuya Tanami.

In July 2015, with help from people affected by leprosy from Brazil who participated in a Papal Mass at Vatican, we delivered a letter to His Holiness. As we received no reply, in November I sent a letter this time to Archbishop Zygmunt Zimowski, president of the Pontifical Council for Health Care Workers—in effect, the Vatican's health minister—requesting his cooperation in convening an international symposium on leprosy, a request I had already made in my letters to the Pope.

For some time this letter elicited no reaction, until 25 January 2016, when I suddenly received a response from Archbishop Zimowski dated 12 January. In it the Archbishop stated that a Year of Mercy had been instituted in December 2015, adding that a Papal Mass "for the sick and persons with disabilities" was scheduled to take place in St. Peter's Square on 12 June 2016. He suggested that the international symposium be convened in conjunction with that event, for two days commencing on 10 June, and he requested that I come to Rome in early February to discuss the matter. I immediately responded with a yes. On the last Sunday of January—World Leprosy Day— Archbishop Zimowski issued a statement on behalf of the Vatican, declaring that an international symposium would be held that June in collaboration with the Nippon Foundation. Not wishing to let this valuable opportunity go by, I immediately decided to send Tatsuya Tanami to Rome.

On 15 February Mr. Tanami was greeted in Rome by various officials of the Pontifical Council for Health Care Workers, including Archbishop

Zimowski and Jean-Marie Mate Musivi Mupendawatu, the organization's secretary. They began the conversation with mention of the close ties that existed between the Vatican's health authority and the Nippon Foundation through the years. Several years earlier, for example, the Pontifical Council had received the Sasakawa Health Prize at the WHO in 1990. And in 2009, the president of the Pontifical Council had been a signatory to that year's Global Appeal to End Stigma and Discrimination against People Affected by Leprosy. We felt honoured that the Council had looked in such detail into these matters.

Archbishop Zimowski clearly wanted the symposium to focus on the human aspect of leprosy, rather than on the disease itself. What is most important, he added, is to strive for the social rehabilitation of persons affected by leprosy and the restoration of their dignity. This being so, he said he wanted the symposium to shed light primarily on those affected by leprosy—which is precisely what we had in mind. He further stressed the overriding importance of restoring the dignity, rights and peace of mind of all those who had ever experienced isolation from society and their home communities.

The Archbishop pointed out that through the years Christian missionaries and other religious affiliates had extended assistance to people suffering from leprosy, and he suggested that they too be invited to the conference to speak of their experiences. We agreed with each other on the basic structure of the symposium and started preparations. We only had four months in which to do this. Then, with full support from the Pontifical Council, the Nippon Foundation contacted potential invitees to the conference, working on the programmes and logistical arrangements at full speed. The Sovereign Order of Malta and Fondation Raoul Follereau were asked to join as co-organizers. We really thought that this was going to be an epoch-making event in which religious leaders and people affected by leprosy would meet and exchange views.

For many years I had harboured some doubts about what religions have done for the benefit of people affected with leprosy. Leprosy has been an affliction of humankind going back to earliest times. Records of the disease are found in ancient Indian texts from the sixth century BCE, and leprosy appears frequently in the Old Testament. Those afflicted by leprosy are regularly described as "unclean", and their suffering is said to be divine punishment for sins committed against God. They were ostracized by—and forced to live apart from—both their families and their "camp," i.e. their community. Jesus, however, extended the hand of salvation and is recorded as having cured persons with the disease, and this was taken as a sign that Jesus was indeed the long-awaited Messiah. Yet despite this all, leprosy itself—the disease—was not done away with.

In Europe during the Middle Ages, anyone who was found to have leprosy was considered dead, and a "Mass of Separation" was conducted for the "deceased" in church. The "deceased" person was then placed in a shelter built by the church expressly for this purpose. In AD 1220, a total of some 19,000 shelters of this kind are said to have existed in Europe. Persons afflicted with leprosy were forced to wear special clothing, to ring a bell to let others know of their presence, and to use a cane to indicate what they wanted. They were cared for by religious orders, even though they were regarded as outcasts.

In Japan, too, it was religious leaders—in this case, Buddhist leaders—who devoted themselves to saving leprosy patients. The earliest record is found in *Nihon Shoki*, an eighth-century chronicle of Japanese history. In the eyes of the leaders of Buddhism, leprosy was a disease visited upon a human being as punishment for a transgression committed by a family relation in a former life—a notion common throughout the world. In Japan, the immediate family of a leprosy patient and any blood relations were subjected to special treatment: exclusion from their community. Meanwhile, Buddhist leaders demonstrated mercy toward leprosy patients and cared for them in order to save their souls, a point in common with Christianity.

In Islam too, leprosy was something to be feared. Believers were urged never to go near a leprosy patient. Generally therefore, religions—all religions—put effort into saving leprosy patients, but the patients nonetheless were separated from their communities, isolated, and treated as dead: actions that no doubt added fuel to the flames of social stigma and discrimination. Against this historical backdrop, I was immensely pleased that the Vatican had accepted our proposal to hold this international symposium and I was eager to see how the issues surrounding leprosy in contemporary times would be addressed and debated.

On 8 June, prior to the conference, there was a Papal Mass held in St. Peter's Square. I was invited to have a seat in the front row where I could meet and speak directly to the Pope. I was told that I should be in my place two hours before the Mass started. Waiting in the strong sunshine, I put my jacket over my head to avoid getting sunburned. Eventually the Mass started and after long prayers the Pope moved around in an open car sending his blessings to the faithful. Some of the people were in tears. Then the Pope alighted from the car and walked to us. When he reached me, I handed over a photo of my father taken with Pope John Paul II and a sheet of paper with a message in Italian saying, "Please do not use leprosy as a negative metaphor." The Pope smiled, took the paper and left. I felt as if I had accomplished a huge task by being able to plead directly with the Pope, and it left me exhausted. I thought it must have been rare indeed for a lay person to deliver such a candid request to the Pope personally.

The symposium took place on 9 and 10 June 2016, one day earlier than originally proposed. In all, some 250 individuals from 45 countries participated, including religious leaders, members of the United Nations Human Rights Council Advisory Committee, medical experts, NGO affiliates, members of the general public, and people affected by leprosy. Of the religious leaders, clergy representing the Catholic Church, Judaism, Islam, Hinduism and Buddhism presented their various interpretations of leprosy and ways of caring for those affected by it.

The core proceedings opened with a presentation by a cardinal representing the Vatican. He related how the Church has historically sought to provide merciful care for leprosy patients, persons who were seen as unclean and recipients of divine punishment, citing such examples as Jesus Christ, Francis of Assisi, Father Damien, and Mother Teresa. The speech given by the representative of Islam made an especially deep impression on me. He said Islam teaches that all sick persons should be treated with merciful kindness, adding that the Quran itself states that such persons should be given succour and their ties with their families should never be put asunder. His words renewed my hopes for the role fulfilled by religion.

Also taking to the podium were people affected by leprosy representing India, Brazil, Ghana, China, Korea, the Philippines, Colombia and Japan. They shared their life histories and the initiatives being taken to eliminate discrimination. Masao Ishida, a resident of Nagashima Aiseien, a former leprosarium in Japan's Inland Sea, spoke of how he had been involuntarily sequestered there upon contracting leprosy at the age of 10. He recalled the situation in those early postwar times: how leprosy had then become curable with the emergence of promin, reviving his awareness of his human rights and spurring his participation, together with fellow inmates, in the movement to abolish Japan's Leprosy Prevention Law. Mr. Ishida continued by describing his current activities and goals. He was then working to get Japan's National Hansen's Disease Museum and affiliated institutes added to UNESCO's Memory of the World register. "It's hard work," he said, "but we believe it is our mission to carry on, backed by our firm conviction that that cruel and miserable history must never be repeated." The way Mr. Ishida approaches his life's duty and the initiatives he is pursuing surely gave great encouragement to the people affected by leprosy in countries where unjustifiable discrimination and practices remain.

The symposium closed on 10 June with a presentation of "Conclusions and Recommendations" based on the issues raised and testimonies given over the course of the two days. The speaker pointed out that, owing to the prejudice and discriminatory practices still prevalent among the public, the human rights of people affected by leprosy and their family members have still not been fully secured. And he averred that representatives of the world's religions must play a vital role toward eliminating such prejudice and discrimination. It was also suggested that use of words that fuel prejudice—especially use of the term "leper"—should henceforth be avoided.

On the day after the symposium, 11 June, a session was held with people affected by leprosy and members of the UN Human Rights Council Advisory Committee. The session had been organized in order to convey the situation of leprosy-related discrimination in countries everywhere, to enable the Committee to understand the extent to which the principles and guidelines for eliminating discrimination against leprosy have taken root around the world. It was significant in allowing the voices of people affected by leprosy to be heard directly by experts in human rights as they described the issues they confronted and the initiatives being taken in their respective countries. All the participants in the meeting were greatly roused by the statements made by a participant from Colombia. "The measures taken by the government have made no progress," he declared. "If discrimination is to be eliminated, it's us who have to take the lead and move into action."

On 12 June, a Sunday, we attended a special Holy Mass—the Jubilee for the Sick and Persons with Disabilities—in St. Peter's Square, a papal event titled Extraordinary Jubilee of Mercy. The event drew roughly seventy thousand people. They listened closely to the words spoken by the Pope. From early morning, Rome was visited by a steady light rain, but just before the Mass was to begin, the rain came to a sudden halt and the skies cleared. I was deeply moved, certain that this was a sign that the Mass and symposium both had God's blessing.

During the Mass, Pope Francis told the crowd that an international conference on leprosy had just been held in Rome in conjunction with the Jubilee for the Sick and Persons with Disabilities, and with gratitude he welcomed the conference organizers and participants. He said that he sincerely hoped that the initiatives taken to fight this disease would bear much fruit, whereupon great applause erupted from the audience. The people affected by leprosy from South America and the Philippines, which are home to large numbers of Roman Catholics, appeared to be particularly moved by the Pope's words. I felt that this message from the Vatican—the Holy See for some 1.2 billion Roman Catholics all around the world—urging elimination of discrimination against leprosy, would surely have a great impact on global society. It marked a giant step forward.

I hope and pray that initiatives taken by the world's religions will greatly strengthen efforts to eliminate discrimination against those affected by leprosy.

AFTERWORD

I have been working for a world without leprosy for more than four decades, often spending a third of each year overseas.

I was born the third son of Ryoichi Sasakawa, who was depicted in the media as a "right-wing heavyweight," an "accused Class A war criminal," and a "freewheeling manipulator of the proceeds from the motorboat racing industry." The reason why I chose to make the elimination of leprosy and the restoration of Ryoichi Sasakawa's reputation my life's work is that I felt the discrimination against persons affected by leprosy as well as against my father was unwarranted and outrageous. I believed it was my destiny and mission to right this injustice.

Seeing my father offering encouragement to a person with a disability or hugging someone seriously disfigured by leprosy, I really sensed his very deep affection for his fellow human beings. I was also immensely impressed by his foresight in utilizing proceeds from gambling on motorboat racing to develop various non-profit activities in the public interest. He was a pioneer in channeling the forces of the private sector to contribute to the public good.

This January 2019 I turned 80 years old. However, I remain confident in my mental and physical abilities and intend to devote all my energies for the rest of my days to reach the goal I have set for myself, which is to realize a leprosy-free world.

This volume was first published in Japanese as *Zanshin* by Gentosha in 2014. Some updates and additions have been made for publication in English. I have received help and support from numerous individuals in Japan and abroad. In particular, I would like to express my gratitude to the staff of the Nippon Foundation and the Sasakawa Health Foundation, who have worked with me for the elimination of leprosy worldwide. I would also like to thank the translator, Rei Muroji, and Hurst Publishers. Last but not least, I would like to thank my wife, Kazuyo, from the bottom of my heart, for her dedication to me and our family.

May 1, 2019
Yohei Sasakawa

INDEX

213

INDEX

INDEX

INDEX

INDEX

INDEX

INDEX

INDEX

INDEX

INDEX